7/20

EMERGENCY
FIRST AID

For Your Cat

Tamara S. Shearer, D.V.M.
Edited by Stanford Apseloff

EMERGENCY FIRST AID

For Your Cat

Tamara S. Shearer, D.V.M.
Edited by Stanford Apseloff

OHIO DISTINCTIVE PUBLISHING
Columbus, Ohio 1995

Published by Ohio Distinctive Publishing, Inc.
4588 Kenny Rd., Columbus OH 43220
www.ohio-distinctive.com

Printed in the United States of America.

97   8 7 6 5 4 3

Illustrated by Claudia Beth Sheets

ISBN: 0-9647934-1-5

Library of Congress Catalog Card Number: 95-71696

This book is dedicated to
my patients
and
cats everywhere.

Special thanks to Stan

ABOUT THE AUTHOR

Dr. Tamara Shearer owns and operates a small-animal veterinary practice in Columbus, Ohio and teaches a cat and dog first-aid course. She is on the Board of Directors of the Columbus Veterinary Emergency Service and is a member of the Citizens for Humane Action Animal Shelter, the American Veterinary Medical Association and the Ohio Veterinary Medical Association. Dr. Shearer has appeared as a veterinary medical advisor on local television and is a university guest lecturer and guest practitioner. Dr. Shearer has a Doctor of Veterinary Medicine degree from The Ohio State University College of Veterinary Medicine and is licensed to practice veterinary medicine in Ohio and California. She is one of the few veterinarians who still make house calls. Dr. Shearer owns fourteen cats.

TABLE OF CONTENTS

PART 1 - GETTING STARTED

Special Comments / 6

Introduction / 7

Prevention / 8

The First-Aid Kit / 14

How To Approach An Emergency / 17

Restraint / 19

Transportation / 23

Special Considerations / 26

PART 2 - FIRST-AID TECHNIQUES

Introduction to Techniques / 30

Bleeding Control / 31

Wound Care / 33

Wrapping a Wound / 35

Monitoring Vital Signs / 37

Inducing Vomiting / 39

Cardiopulmonary Resuscitation / 40

How to Make a Cat Muzzle / 44

Elizabethan Collar / 47

PART 3 - HELP FOR THE PROBLEM

Introductory Information / 52

Problem/Condition (Listed Alphabetically) / 53

Symptoms (Listed Alphabetically) / 134

PART 4 - POISON BASICS

General Procedures / 176
List of Common Poisons / 178

PART 5 - POISONOUS PLANTS

Introduction to Poisonous Plants / 182
Poisonous Plants (Listed Alphabetically) / 183
Plants that Cause Skin Irritation / 231
Nonpoisonous Plants / 232

PART 6 - OTHER POISONS

Other Poisons (Listed Alphabetically) / 234

PART 7 - DISEASES THAT CAN BECOME EMERGENCIES

General Information / 260
Dental Disease / 261
Infections / 263
Cancers / 265
Long-Term Illnesses / 267
Skin Irritations / 269
Soft Stools/Diarrhea / 270
Intestinal Parasites / 272
External Parasites (Listed Alphabetically) / 274

PART 8 - MISCELLANEOUS

Deliveries / 282
Raising Orphan Kittens / 285
False Emergencies / 288
The Hospitalized Cat / 290
The Lost Cat / 292

APPENDICES

Lost Pet Information / 296
Medical Health Record / 297
Emergency Worksheet / 299
Normal Vital Signs for Cats / 300
Preventive Health Care / 301
Physical Examination / 305

BIBLIOGRAPHY / 311

INDEX / 313

PART 1

—

GETTING STARTED

SPECIAL COMMENTS

This book is a first-aid guide for common emergencies. It is meant to be used as an aid when immediate veterinary care is unavailable. This book should not be used as a substitute for veterinary care. Because your veterinarian will be able to advise you best based on the particular circumstances of your cat's emergency, you should contact your veterinarian at the earliest possible moment, preferably before initiating any nonessential treatment.

INTRODUCTION

It was New Year's Eve, and the Andersons were enjoying the night's festivities, as was Oscar, the family feline. Oscar feasted on the newest addition to the windowsill plant family, a bright red poinsettia. By the time someone noticed, the poinsettia looked distressed, and so did Oscar.

This book is designed to teach cat owners, like the Andersons, how to tend to their pet's medical emergencies until they can get professional veterinary assistance. By using the emergency first-aid guidance provided by this book, you can learn to recognize a medical emergency and treat it appropriately.

This book will discuss how to handle the injured or sick cat, how to make a first-aid kit, how to assess an emergency situation, and how to treat your pet during a crisis. This book provides instruction for treating a host of problems ranging from minor ailments to severe situations, including bite wounds, poisoning and being hit by a car.

PREVENTION

The best way to remedy an emergency is to prevent it from happening. By recognizing potential hazards before they occur, you may save your cat's life. Cats are curious by nature and are adept at finding trouble. Because of the number of hazards outdoors, cats should, ideally, be confined to the house. Outdoor cats can explore dangerous places, and when they do get into trouble, you might not be there to help. Also, with outdoor cats it is difficult to monitor attitude, appetite, toilet habits and other behavior for signs of illness; many seriously ill or injured outdoor cats seek out hiding places and often die.

Because indoor cats are often masters of escape, owners should, as a precaution, provide their cats with identification, regardless of whether the pets are permitted outdoors. The identification should be in the form of a tag that includes the owner's name, address, and telephone number on one side and the veterinarian's name, address and telephone number on the opposite side. Proper identification is important in facilitating treatment. If a pet is away from its home and an illness or injury occurs, the owner can be identified and notified of the situation. The identification tag should directly adhere to the pet's collar and should not be left dangling. A dangling tag can become stuck in and on various objects and pose some risk. (However, any identification is better than none.) Also, to prevent injury, the collar should be the type that will permit the cat to slip out of it if the collar gets caught on something.

Outdoor cats have more exposure than indoor cats to poisons, and outdoor cats risk a multitude of traumas, including injury from cars, guns, other animals and even people. Outside cats also have a higher risk of getting infections because of their increased exposure to disease. Infections like panleukopenia (distemper), feline leukemia, feline infectious peritonitis and feline immunosuppressive virus can be fatal. Parasitic infections can also cause serious disease.

Both indoor and outdoor cats may be at risk of trauma from what is commonly called "high-rise syndrome". Cats like to perch on high places, such as the window sill in a high-rise apartment or the edge of a high balcony. Although they act as though they are in no danger, many cats eventually fall or jump from their perches and sustain serious injuries. Note that screens in windows may not be enough of a barrier to prevent your cat from falling out of a window; keep windows above the ground floor at least partially closed to protect your cat from an accident.

Outdoor precautions include providing the cat with fresh food and water. (Note that water may freeze quickly in the winter months.) In the cool months, the cat should have good shelter away from drafts and dampness. When the temperature falls below freezing, all outdoor cats should be moved inside or provided with an alternative heat source like a heat lamp. Their paws should be kept clean of ice, salt and mud. Because trapping is a cool weather sport, in the winter months you should check nearby creek beds for pets that have become accidentally caught in leg-hold traps.

In the summer months, it is particularly important that outdoor cats have access to plenty of fresh water. Also, they should have adequate shade from summer mid-day heat. If your cat spends time in a shed or garage, good ventilation is essential.

Because outdoor cats have a tendency to eat grass, it is important to keep your cat indoors if your lawn has been chemically treated recently with pesticides or fertilizers. Lawn chemicals can poison a cat, or they may cause chemical burns to the pet's feet. Also, if you have recently sprayed insecticides inside your home, keep your cat out of the rooms that have been sprayed until the chemicals dissipate.

Even though indoor cats live in a more sheltered environment, they too are not without risk. Modifying their environment can help decrease the likelihood of emergencies. Cat-proof your home by removing potential hazards. Make sure electrical and other cords are not dangling in a manner that will entice your cat to play with them. Electrical cords can cause severe burns or death if your cat chews through the protective insulation, and any type of cord (e.g., telephone, drapery, etc.) poses a danger of strangulation. Also, keep your indoor cat's claws well-trimmed to prevent them from catching on carpets, draperies and furniture.

Cats love to play with and chew small items such as paper clips, staples, rubber bands, pins, buttons, trash-bag ties, Christmas-tree tinsel, yarn and string. These objects, once swallowed, cannot be digested and cannot pass through the bowels; the result is often lethal unless the object is surgically removed. As a precaution, you should remove all strings from any of your cat's toys, and make sure your cat never plays with yarn or string of any kind. Keep a close inventory of your stationery supplies (rubber bands, paper clips, staples, tacks, etc.), and make sure they are stored in a secure location. Never decorate a Christmas tree with tinsel if your cat has any chance of getting to the tree because tinsel is extremely destructive to a cat's digestive system, and even a small amount can be fatal.

Toxic indoor plants should be identified and removed or kept out of reach. (See Part 5 - Poisonous Plants.) If your cat is permitted outside, to the extent possible you should attempt to limit its access to potentially harmful plants.

Never use a flea product on cats if it is labeled for dogs only. Flea dips for dogs can be especially dangerous for cats. Also, flea products for cats can become toxic when not used properly. Always read and follow product labels carefully.

Never feed your cat chocolate, table scraps or bones. Chocolate is poisonous to cats because it contains theobromine, which they cannot metabolize. In general, table scraps can predispose the cat to pancreatitis and other digestive upsets, and milk can be a major cause of diarrhea. Bones cannot be digested and can pierce the digestive-tract lining, possibly causing fatal peritonitis (inflammation within the abdomen). As a preventive measure, keep all people food away from your cat, and keep trash containers secured.

People medications are often poisonous to cats. Aspirin, acetaminophen (Tylenol®) and ibuprofen are all potentially lethal for felines. (See pages 63, 56 and 97.) Never administer medications of any type without specific instructions from your veterinarian.

Finally, make sure your cat is up-to-date on its vaccinations. The appendix section on Preventive Health Care lists the vaccinations that your cat should receive as well as a timetable for both vaccinations and boosters. Many cat diseases that are easily preventable with a vaccine are incurable, including rabies which can be transmitted to people.

The reasonable precautions discussed above and outlined below should decrease the risk of an emergency and may save your cat's life.

I. Accident-Proofing your Home

A. Keep telephone cords, drapery cords and electrical cords out of reach.

B. Pick up small nondigestible objects: paper clips, pins, rubber bands, staples, needles, thread, yarn, string, etc.

C. Make sure that your cat toys do not have any string or yarn as part of the toy.

D. Do not decorate a Christmas tree with tinsel.

E. Keep your indoor cat's claws trimmed.

F. Never give your cat human medications of any kind without specific instructions from a veterinarian. Aspirin, acetaminophen (Tylenol®) and ibuprofen can be fatal to your cat. Keep all medications out of your cat's reach.

G. Identify and remove toxic plants and flowers. (Refer to the Poisonous Plants chapter of this book.)

H. Keep your cat off of lawns that have been recently treated with pesticides or fertilizers.

I. Keep your cat out of rooms where you have recently sprayed indoor insecticides.

J. Never use snail bait, rat poison or poisonous ant traps.

K. Never use continual-release toilet disinfectants.

L. Keep your clothes-dryer door closed.

M. Keep windows above the ground floor at least partially closed.

N. Provide good ventilation during hot summer months.

O. Keep all trash containers covered.

II. Prevention for Outside the Home

A. Provide your cat with an identification tag.

B. Properly dispose of antifreeze.

C. Never use snail bait or rat poison.

D. Secure openings in outdoor air-conditioning units.

E. Honk horn before starting your car engine.

F. Honk your car horn before pulling out of the driveway.

G. Identify and remove toxic plants and flowers. (Refer to the Poisonous Plants chapter in this book.)

H. In the winter, provide fresh water, and change it before it freezes.
I. In cool months, provide dry, draft-free shelter.
J. During hot summer months, provide well-ventilated shelter.

III. Preventive Medicine

A. Keep vaccinations and physical exams up to date.
B. Follow flea-product instructions carefully.
C. Never give any medication without a veterinarian's advice.
D. Never give your cat any people medications like aspirin, acetaminophen (Tylenol®) or ibuprofen – these substances can be deadly.
E. Spay or neuter your cat.

IV. Additional Measures

A. Keep your cat inside, if possible.
B. Never leave a cat alone for an extended period of time.
C. Never leave a cat alone in a hot car with the windows up.
D. Do not declaw an outdoor cat.
E. Keep hair coat free of mats (to prevent skin sores).
F. Keep paws free of ice, mud and salt; wash and dry the paws.

V. Preventive Nutrition

A. Never feed cats dog food. The lack of the protein taurine in dog food can cause blindness and heart failure in cats. Dog foods also lack other nutrients essential for healthy cats.

B. Never feed cats milk. Milk can cause digestive problems like diarrhea.

C. Do not supplement diets without a veterinarian's advice. Wrong supplementation can cause urinary tract problems, metabolic problems and even mineralization of the kidneys.

D. Never feed a cat raw fish. Raw fish causes a thiamine deficiency which may result in loss of appetite, a hunched and painful stance and possibly convulsions.

E. Never feed a cat a diet of fish exclusively. Fish, even when cooked, can cause a vitamin E deficiency leading to inflammation of fatty tissue (causing pain when the cat moves or is touched), fever and a reluctance to move.

F. Never feed a cat foods high in magnesium; it may predispose the cat to urinary tract problems. Consult your veterinarian for specific recommendations.

G. Never feed your cat table scraps, bones or chocolates.

THE FIRST-AID KIT

The most important feature of a first-aid kit is accessibility. The kit must be readily available when an emergency occurs. Therefore, it is important to keep the kit in a location that is obvious (e.g., beside the cat food) and in a location that provides easy access, such as an unlocked drawer or cupboard. The items in a kit should be kept within a container that is easily transported, in case you need to bring the kit to the cat. Finally, the kit should be in a closed container that will keep its contents clean and dry. A fishing tackle or utility box would be a good choice.

Once you have selected a suitable container for the kit, it is time to stock it with the items you will most likely need in an emergency. First, stock your kit with three large plastic garbage bags to protect car upholstery and household furnishings from blood, urine and feces. Then include 2 rolls of 3" gauze bandage and 12 gauze sponges 3"x3" for wound care. Obtain adhesive tape of the nonstick type; it will provide more comfort to your cat than ordinary tape that sticks to fur. Next, add scissors and toenail trimmers, several paper towels (for cleaning up messes), antibiotic ointment, saline solution (the kind people use for contact-lens cleaning), tweezers, an eyedropper (for use in force-feeding liquid medications), a rectal thermometer, nonstick bandages, alcohol and hydrogen peroxide. Also include a cat muzzle, preferably the nylon variety as opposed to a leather one. A nylon muzzle is more comfortable for your pet and can be laundered easily. In a pinch you can construct a muzzle from a paper cup and gauze (see page 44 in the First-Aid Techniques section of this book), but a homemade muzzle will be more difficult to use on your cat and may not work as well. If you are going to use a homemade muzzle, make it now; in an emergency, you will have plenty of other things to do.

Other items that are useful but will not fit into your first-aid container should be kept in close proximity to the kit. Make sure you have two 2-liter soda bottles that you can fill with warm water in an emergency to help keep your cat from getting chilled. Also have access to clean bath towels and a blanket to aid in transportation and restraint and to provide warmth. Finally, get a pet carrier so that you can safely transport your pet in an emergency. If you are unable to

14

obtain a pet carrier, make sure you have a ventilated box that is the appropriate size and is suitably durable to serve as a substitute.

To ensure you have easy access to professional help, make a list of telephone numbers of the pet's daytime veterinarian, a reserve day-time veterinarian, two night-time veterinary emergency numbers, the local poison control hotline, and the National Animal Poison Control Center. (The National Animal Poison Control Center provides assistance for a fee - $20 for 5 minutes at the time of this printing: 1-900-680-0000.) Put one copy of the list in your first-aid kit and another near the telephone.

I. First-Aid Box

A. Obtain a box that is
    (1) Transportable (shoe-box size, preferably with a handle)
    (2) Durable and water-resistant (like a fishing tackle box)
    (3) Non-locking (to provide easy access).
B. Label the outside of the box "CAT FIRST AID".
C. Store the first-aid box in plain view.

II. First-Aid Provisions (to put into First-Aid Box)

A. 3 large garbage bags
B. 2 rolls of 3" gauze bandage
C. 12 gauze sponges 3" x 3"
D. Nonstick adhesive tape
E. Scissors
F. Nail trimmers
G. Antibiotic ointment (e.g., Polysporin®) – small tube
H. Saline solution – 8 ounces (same as used for contact-lens care)
I. Hydrogen peroxide – 8 ounces
J. Muzzle – preferably nylon
K. Rectal thermometer

L. Alcohol
M. Tweezers
N. Eyedropper
O. Nonstick bandages
P. Water-soluble lubricating jelly (e.g., K-Y™ Brand)
Q. Paper towels – to clean up any mess
R. Emergency information (see below)

III. Emergency Information

A. Emergency telephone numbers:
   (1) Poison control _____
   (2) Veterinarians _____

   _____
   (3) After-hours veterinarians_____

   _____
   (4) Fire department _____
B. A copy of this book
C. A copy of the First-Aid Provisions List
D. A plant identification book

IV. Additional First-Aid Items

A. Towels – for use in restraining your cat
B. Blanket – to keep your cat warm and comfortable
C. Pet carrier – to transport your cat
D. Two 2-liter soda bottles – for use as hot-water bottles

HOW TO APPROACH AN EMERGENCY

When an emergency occurs, the first step is to decide whether to become involved. Evaluate the risk to you, the cat and others. Be conscious of the surroundings. For example, if you are driving and you see an injured cat at the side of the highway, first consider whether there is a safe place to stop, and then consider whether the situation could get worse if the cat runs when you try to approach it. If the overall risk is too great, then do not become involved.

Pet emergencies are stressful, and your anxiety can interfere with your common sense. It is important to stay as calm as possible during an emergency in order to give your cat the best care. If you become too emotional, it may be advisable to have a family member or friend help provide care. Remember that your pet is totally dependent upon you during an emergency.

One of the most important actions you can take prior to an emergency is to make arrangements to have access to veterinary care 24 hours a day. This may take some planning, especially if you live in a rural area. Most large cities have pet emergency-care centers. Even though the pet may have a regular veterinarian, it is a good idea to have at least one other doctor available as a backup during the day. Also, make arrangements to have two night-time veterinarians available. In selecting your emergency veterinary numbers, it is important for you to consider not only the skills of the veterinarians but also their locations. The closer the doctor's office, the better the pet's chances if a problem occurs in which time is a factor. The veterinarians' telephone numbers should be listed near the phone as well as in your first-aid kit.

Make sure any pet sitter understands the emergency instructions. The pet sitter should know whom to contact in case of an emergency. The cat's doctor should also be notified of treatment preferences in the event of an emergency when the owner is unavailable; otherwise the veterinarian will likely provide only basic care until given permission to proceed with additional treatments.

Regardless of the emergency, there are some basic steps that you can take to help your cat. The following information should enable you to take appropriate action in a wide variety of emergency situations.

17

I. Basic Steps in Emergency Care

A. Stay calm. Focus on the cat's needs. Use common sense during the crisis. If you are unable to deal with the situation, then delegate the emergency care to someone else.

B. Observe the urgency. Does the emergency appear to be mild, moderate, or severe? Evaluate whether the situation is getting better, staying the same, or getting worse.

C. Seek assistance:
   (1) Call the cat's doctor.
   (2) If the emergency occurs outside of regular veterinary hours, call for after-hour help.
   (3) If you suspect poisoning and cannot reach a veterinarian, call your local poison control hotline or the National Animal Poison Control Center. (The National Animal Poison Control Center provides assistance for a fee – $20 for 5 minutes at the time of this printing: 1-900-680-0000.)
   (4) If no professional help is available, proceed to Step II.

II. First-Aid Instructions

A. Identify the problem or symptom; then refer to the alphabetically-arranged emergency section or to the index of this book.

B. If the problem cannot be identified, follow these steps:
   (1) Confine the cat.
   (2) Keep the cat quiet and warm.
   (3) Note any and all symptoms.
   (4) Observe whether the condition is getting better, staying the same or getting worse.

C. Contact a veterinarian as soon as possible.

RESTRAINT

Hurt or sick pets may react unpredictably; often instinctual behavior overrides normal disposition. This is important to remember when your pet needs special handling or treatment during an emergency. Cats usually respond to illness in one of three ways: some will not show behavioral changes and will respond to handling in their normal manner; others may become listless or depressed, in which case they tend to be relatively easy to handle; and others may become anxious or aggressive, an instinctive reaction often associated with pain and fear. This instinctive reaction can make handling and treatment very difficult. When an anxious cat struggles, it poses a risk of injury to the caretaker; a scared cat will often bite and scratch.

Struggling cats also pose a risk of further injuring themselves. In cases where the cat is frightened, is in obvious pain or is behaving aggressively, your approach and handling techniques are important. Approach an anxious or aggressive cat slowly and calmly, talking quietly to the pet. Some cats respond to repetitive sounds like quiet clicking, purring or kissing noises. If the cat tries to flee and it is evident that it needs first-aid, your first step is to decide whether to intervene. There is often a risk to both the cat and you in this situation. In addition, an outdoor cat that is not vaccinated may carry rabies, a disease that can be fatal to people. If you make the decision not to intervene, you may wish to employ the help of a professional such as a house-call veterinarian or a humane-society volunteer. These professionals are proficient at dealing with hard-to-handle cats.

If you decide to intervene, manual restraint of a cat can be accomplished by approaching from behind and grabbing the scruff of the cat's neck (i.e., the skin and soft tissue on the back of the cat's neck). See illustration on page 21. Always approach a pet from behind to avoid being bitten or scratched. Once the cat is in hand, the pet can be lifted or positioned for further care or examination. See illustration on page 22. If the cat is fighting, this method of restraint may cause risk of injury, and you should consider using a large towel, blanket or fish net instead of your hands. Slowly approach the pet (from behind, if possible) and place the towel, blanket or net over the cat. If a fracture, neck or back injury is suspected, take care to avoid excessive movement of the cat. Movement can be minimized by sliding the pet onto a small board or directly into a pet carrier.

If you follow the rules for several basic restraint techniques, the stress during an emergency will be decreased for the pet and for you.

I. Behavioral Changes Affecting Restraint of the Sick, Hurt Cat

A. Listless or depressed cats may be easier to handle.
B. Hurt or sick cats may become anxious or aggressive and be more difficult to handle. They may scratch or bite.
C. Some cats may not show behavioral changes and may be predictable to handle.

II. Approaching an Injured Cat

A. Talk to the cat calmly and quietly.
B. Move toward the cat slowly.
C. Do not chase the cat.

III. Restraining a Depressed or Easy-to-Handle Cat

A. Approach from behind to prevent getting bitten or scratched.
B. Gather the skin of the scruff of the neck in one hand.
C. Lift the cat gently by the scruff while supporting the hind legs.
D. If the cat needs to be held stationary, push down gently at the shoulders while holding the scruff.

IV. Restraining the Hard-to-Handle Cat

A. Obtain a towel, blanket, net, heavy leather gloves and a muzzle.
B. Approach from behind to help prevent getting bitten.
C. If the cat is trying to bite, use a muzzle. (See pages 44 to 46.)
D. If the cat is trying to scratch, wear heavy leather gloves.
Caution: cats can bite through virtually any gloves!
E. Place the towel, blanket or net over the cat.
F. Gather the cat in the towel, blanket or net to complete the restraint.

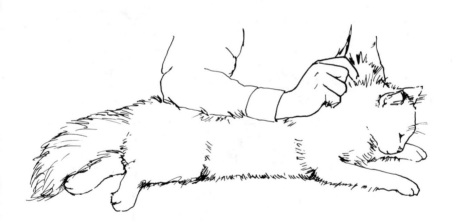

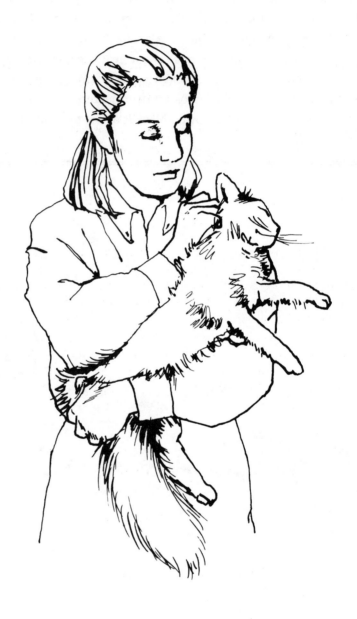

TRANSPORTATION

Transporting an injured cat can sometimes be as stressful and as hazardous to the cat as the emergency itself. Most cats do not like riding in cars, but even those who do not generally mind the experience may act differently under emergency conditions. A cat who is naturally docile may revert to instinctive reactions and become frantic. In addition to distracting you from your driving, an unrestricted cat in the car may crawl onto or under the gas or brake pedal or may crawl up into the dashboard to hide.

A pet carrier is the preferred method of transport, although a sturdy corrugated box with small air holes may suffice in an emergency. When selecting a pet carrier, choose one that is spacious enough for the cat to be comfortable. The medium-sized carriers are generally preferable. Cardboard carriers are not as sturdy as plastic ones, and some cats can escape from the cardboard carriers by clawing or biting through the box. A plastic carrier with a removable top is ideal because it enables you to put the cat into or remove the cat from the carrier without having to push or pull the animal.

It is important to note that the cat's condition will dictate the specific procedures that you will need to use for safe transport. The outline that follows is a guide to transport under a variety of emergency conditions.

I. Equipment Needed in Transportation

A. Plastic or cardboard cat carrier
B. Towel
C. Blanket
D. 2-liter soda bottle filled with warm water
E. Muzzle
F. Collar and leash

II. Transporting a Cat in Stable Condition

A. Line a carrier with a towel.

B. If the cat is hard to handle, you may wish to use a muzzle. However, use a muzzle only if the cat is not having difficulty breathing and has not been vomiting. If at any time the cat has difficulty breathing, remove the muzzle.

C. Put the cat in the carrier. (If the cat is hesitant to enter the carrier head first, back the cat into the carrier.)

D. Close the carrier door quickly.

III. Transporting a Cat in Shock

A. Place a towel in the carrier.

B. Place the cat in the carrier.

C. Place a 2-liter soda bottle filled with warm water (not hot water) into the carrier beside the cat. See illustration on page 111.

D. Make sure the water bottle keeps the cat warm but does not burn the pet.

IV. Transporting a Cat with Fractures or Back Injuries

A. Place a towel in the carrier.

B. Place a 2-liter soda bottle filled with warm water wrapped with a towel into the carrier.

C. If the cat is not having difficulty breathing and has not been vomiting, carefully place a muzzle on the cat prior to moving the animal. If at any time the cat has difficulty breathing or acts nauseous, remove the muzzle.

D. Avoid excess movement of the cat. Movement can be minimized by sliding the pet onto a small board or directly into a pet carrier.

E. To minimize discomfort, transport with the fractured side up.

V. Transporting a Cat Without a Pet Carrier

A. Alternative equipment
  (1) 2 clothes baskets
  (2) Heavy cardboard box and tape
  (3) Collar and leash
B. Transportation using 2 clothes baskets
  (1) Place a towel in one basket.
  (2) Place the cat in the basket.
  (3) Place the other basket upside down on top of the bottom one, and secure them together using tape or gauze tied through the holes.
C. Transportation using a heavy cardboard box
  (1) Place a towel in the box.
  (2) Cut three to five small 1/2 inch holes in the box.
  (3) Place the cat in the box.
  (4) Tape the box securely by wrapping tape around the full dimension of the box.
D. Transportation using a collar and leash.
  (1) Place a collar with a leash around the pet's neck.
  (2) Wrap the cat in a towel.
  (3) Get someone to hold the cat while it is being transported.

SPECIAL CONSIDERATIONS

"Special considerations" refers to conditions that may complicate emergency treatment. In particular, this chapter will address the special needs of kittens, older cats and cats with preexisting diseases or medical conditions. Because each cat has unique characteristics, you should consult your veterinarian regarding any special treatment or special considerations in the day-to-day care of your pet as well as in emergency situations.

Because of the vast number of special considerations and the unique characteristics of each cat, this chapter can only begin to address the particular needs of your pet. If you suspect that your cat has special needs, find out now before an emergency develops so that you can administer the best possible care for your pet.

I. Kittens

A. Because of a kitten's small body size, it has little reserve to support itself during an illness.
B. Kittens have immature immune systems that are inadequate for fighting infections after the kittens are weaned from their mothers. Make sure your kitten gets timely vaccinations.
C. Because of a kitten's curiosity, it is prone to finding trouble that can result in injury.

II. Older Cats

A. Older cats require special care because their organs/internal functions may be diseased or show aging changes making them more sensitive to disease processes.

B. Make sure older cats have easy access to food and water.

C. Some older cats are prone to becoming underweight; therefore, they have less body reserve than fit cats.

D. Other older cats are overweight, which can predispose them to diseases and slow their recoveries.

E. Cats over 7-8 years of age should have annual blood tests to screen for early diseases of the internal organs, diabetes and anemias. X-rays and an EKG may be warranted to identify early heart disease.

III. Preexisting Diseases

A. Obesity may predispose a cat to early heart, liver and kidney disease. It may also cause problems with urinary-tract irritations and early arthritis.

B. Feline immunosuppressive virus (FIV) and feline leukemia may predispose your cat to other diseases, postpone recovery and/or cause death. In some cases the cat may be a carrier of the disease but not show any symptoms.

C. Metabolic disease problems (e.g., thyroid disorders, diabetes) can complicate recoveries if the diseases are not properly diagnosed and treated.

PART 2

—

FIRST-AID TECHNIQUES

INTRODUCTION TO TECHNIQUES

There are many techniques that you should practice and learn now so that you will know them in the event of an emergency. Repetition and mental preparation will enable you to cope with the stress of an emergency in a more organized manner and will enable you to perform necessary techniques more efficiently.

The eight techniques described in this chapter are presented in logical order: external, internal and other. Bleeding control, wound care and wrapping a wound comprise the external techniques. These three techniques are essential elements of emergency treatment for lacerations, abrasions, bite wounds and a variety of other traumas. Monitoring vital signs (i.e., temperature, pulse and respiration), inducing vomiting and performing cardiopulmonary resuscitation are the three techniques that involve a cat's internal systems. Monitoring vital signs serves in both diagnosis of a problem as well as in the evaluation of severity and change in condition. Inducing vomiting is a procedure that applies to a multitude of situations involving poisoning; it is, in many circumstances, a life-saving technique. Cardiopulmonary resuscitation (CPR) is a technique used in the most critical situations when your cat has stopped breathing and has no pulse. When CPR is necessary, there is no time to find a veterinarian, which means that your ability to perform the technique will determine whether your cat has a chance of surviving.

The two remaining techniques involve construction and use of simple restraining devices: the muzzle and the Elizabethan collar. The muzzle is used primarily to facilitate safe handling of the pet (i.e., to prevent the cat from biting you or someone else), whereas the Elizabethan collar is used to keep the pet from licking or biting itself. Both devices are used in a variety of situations, and it is therefore important that you either purchase a commercial variety of each or else use the instructions in this book to construct home-made versions.

BLEEDING CONTROL

Often an emergency involves some type of hemorrhage (i.e., bleeding). The bleeding may be mild, moderate, or severe. Severe hemorrhage may involve the severing of an artery, injury to a large muscle mass, a fracture of a bone, toxicity due to rat poisoning, or internal trauma to an organ. If the blood pools quickly or pumps in spurts, you can assume it is serious. Immediate action is required to prevent shock.

I.   First-Aid Materials

A.   Clean towel
B.   Gauze sponges
C.   Nonstick adhesive tape
D.   Nonstick bandages
E.   Gauze wrap

II.   Technique Instructions

A.   Locate the source of bleeding.
B.   Using a clean towel or gauze sponges, apply firm direct pressure to the wound for 5-10 minutes.
C.   Note how fast the blood pools or if it spurts. Make an observation of the amount of blood loss. (A 10-pound cat has only about 10 ounces of blood.)
D.   A wrap may be applied to the area if hemorrhage has slowed. (See page 35 on Wrapping a Wound.) DO NOT attempt to clean the wound or apply antibiotic ointment because the clot may be disrupted and severe hemorrhage may resume.

III. Emergency Situations Where the Technique Applies

A. Open fractures
B. Bite wound abscesses
C. Abrasions
D. Lacerations
E. Other trauma, such as gunshot wounds

WOUND CARE

Proper cleansing of wounds can facilitate healing and help prevent infection. Many minor wounds can be treated at home, but they should be checked by a veterinarian who may recommend antibiotics.

I.   First-Aid Materials

A.   Saline solution (i.e., contact-lens saline solution)
B.   Mild antibacterial soap
C.   Water-soluble lubricating jelly (e.g., K-Y™ Brand)
D.   Clippers or scissors
E.   Antibiotic ointment (e.g., Polysporin®)

II.   Technique Instructions

A.   Apply water-soluble lubricating jelly to the wound to protect it from the pet's hair.
B.   Using clippers or carefully using scissors, trim the cat's hair from around the wound.
C.   Using water or saline solution, rinse the lubricating jelly from the wound.
D.   If the wound is visibly soiled, rinse it with water until all debris is removed.
E.   Gently scrub the area using antibacterial soap and water. Rinse well with water, then with saline solution if available.
F.   Apply antibiotic ointment. If necessary to keep the wound clean, apply a wrap. (See Wrapping a Wound on page 35.)

III. Emergencies Situations Where the Technique Applies

A. Burns
B. Abrasions
C. Lacerations
D. Bite wounds
E. Other trauma

WRAPPING A WOUND

Wraps should be applied to areas where abrasions or lacerations are present to keep them clean and to prevent the cat from causing further trauma by licking a wound. In many situations where a wrap is needed, an Elizabethan collar may also be necessary. See page 47.

I. First-Aid Materials

A. Antibiotic ointment (e.g., Polysporin®)
B. Saline solution
C. Nonstick adhesive tape
D. Nonstick bandages
E. Gauze wrap

II. Technique Instructions

A. Treat the injury according to the specific instructions provided elsewhere in this book (e.g., Wound Care on page 33).
B. Apply antibiotic ointment over wound.
C. Press nonstick bandage to wound.
D. Secure nonstick bandage to wound by wrapping gauze around the leg or body. The gauze should be pulled snug but not tight. The wrap tightness should not restrict circulation or the cat's breathing.
E. Secure the gauze by applying adhesive tape to the wrap.
F. Monitor the pet for any evidence of swelling to the limb below the wrap. If swelling occurs, then the wrap is too tight and

should be removed immediately. If the cat's breathing is hindered, also remove the wrap.

III. Emergency Situations Where the Technique Applies

A. Abrasions
B. Lacerations
C. Burns
D. Other skin irritations
E. Compound/open fractures

MONITORING VITAL SIGNS (TEMPERATURE, PULSE AND RESPIRATIONS)

Monitoring vital signs gives the veterinarian and pet owner a basis for evaluating the pet's progress during an illness. The techniques for obtaining pulse and respirations are noninvasive, but unfortunately taking the pet's temperature is a procedure that not every cat will tolerate and not every caretaker may feel comfortable performing. The decision to obtain a temperature from a pet should be based on the pet's disposition and the owner's willingness to participate.

I.   First-Aid Materials

A.   Rectal thermometer
B.   Water-soluble lubricating jelly (e.g., K-Y™ Brand) or petroleum jelly
C.   Watch or clock with second hand

II.   Technique Instructions

A.   Taking the temperature:
   (1)   Lubricate a rectal thermometer with water-soluble lubricating jelly or petroleum jelly. Insert the thermometer gently into the cat's rectum approximately 1/2 to 1 inch.
   (2)   Wait 2 minutes, and then remove and read the thermometer.
   (3)   Normal temperature is between 100.5 and 102.5 degrees Fahrenheit.

B. Taking the pulse:
    (1) Lay your hand just behind the cat's shoulder blade on either side of its chest and feel for the heart beat (as illustrated on page 43), or
    (2) Place your hand in the groin area of the cat's abdomen and feel for the femoral pulse.
    (3) Count the beats per minute (e.g., count for 15 seconds and multiply by 4).
    (4) Normal pulse at rest should range from approximately 110 to 140 beats per minute. If the cat has been recently active or is excited, its pulse may be significantly higher.
C. Taking respirations:
    (1) If the cat is lying quietly, watch the chest rise and fall.
    (2) Count the number of breaths the cat takes in a minute.
    (3) Normal resting respiratory rate is approximately 24 to 28 breaths per minute.

III. Emergency Situations Where the Technique Applies

A. Virtually all conditions

INDUCING VOMITING

When a cat ingests a poisonous substance, time is critical, and your ability to induce your cat to vomit may save its life.

NOTE: Vomiting should NEVER be induced if a pet is unconscious or in a stupor. Also never induce vomiting if there is suspicion of ingestion of petroleum distillates, acids or alkalis (e.g., kerosene, gasoline, motor oil, various household cleaning supplies). As a general rule, follow the instructions on the product warning label regarding whether to induce vomiting. If in doubt, call a poison control center, but make sure you act quickly.

I.   First-Aid Materials

A.   Hydrogen peroxide
B.   Eyedropper

II.   Technique Instructions

A.   Induce vomiting only if the cat is conscious. Before proceeding, attempt to contact your veterinarian. If a veterinarian is not immediately available, then feed the cat 1 teaspoon of hydrogen peroxide (mixed with 1 teaspoon milk if available). If the cat will not drink the mixture or if there is no milk available, then force-feed the cat the hydrogen peroxide using an eyedropper.
B.   If vomiting does not occur within 10 minutes, repeat the procedure twice if needed.
C.   Contact a veterinarian as soon as possible.

III.   Emergencies Situations Where the Technique Applies

A.   Most poisonings. (See note above.)

CARDIOPULMONARY RESUSCITATION

Just like in human medicine, cardiopulmonary resuscitation (CPR) for your cat can mean the difference between life and death. This technique may enable a critically-injured cat to survive until it is transported to a veterinary hospital.

CPR is used to revive a cat that is not breathing and has no heartbeat (e.g., from drowning or severe electrical shock). When CPR is needed, it must be performed immediately. Therefore, it is imperative that you be able to assess the need quickly and perform the technique effectively.

Unlike many other emergency techniques, cardiopulmonary resuscitation is performed without any special equipment or materials.

NOTE: CPR is a technique of last resort when the cat shows no signs of life. If there is any evidence that the cat is breathing, do not perform this technique.

I.   Technique Instructions

A.   Lay the cat on its side (and throughout these procedures keep the cat on its side).

B.   Check for breathing by watching the cat's chest rise and fall.

C.   **If the cat is breathing,** proceed no further. Do not use CPR.

D.   **If the cat is not breathing,**

   (1) Establish an airway by removing any debris from the cat's mouth or by moving the tongue from the back of the throat. (See illustration page 41.) Check for breathing by watching the cat's chest rise and fall. If the cat is breathing, proceed no further, and do not use CPR.

   (2) Check for a pulse by placing a hand over the cat's chest just behind the shoulder blade (see illustration on page 43) to feel the heartbeat or by placing a hand in the groin area to feel the femoral pulse.

40

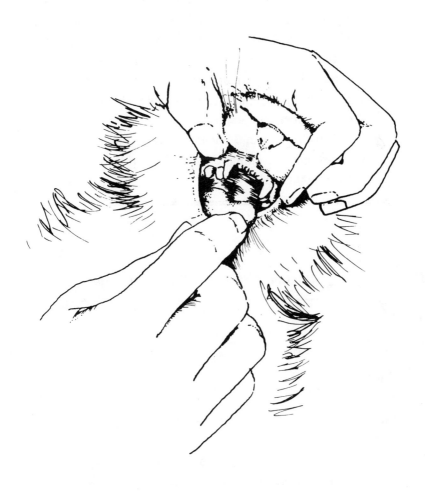

E. **If the cat still is not breathing,**

    (1) Cup your hand(s) over the cat's nose and mouth to form a seal. Deliver 1 breath into the pet every 2 seconds. If the seal is proper, you should observe the cat's chest rise and fall.

    (2) If after you have delivered 5 breaths the cat does not show signs of breathing on its own or signs of consciousness, and there is no heartbeat, then have a helper place a hand just behind the cat's shoulder blades (as illustrated on page 43), and apply gentle but firm compressions downward (compressing 1/2 to 1 inch) at a rate of 1 compression every 2 seconds. If a helper is not available, alternate delivering 2 breaths then 10 compressions.

    (3) Check for a pulse and breathing every 2 minutes. If there is no pulse and breathing, continue for up to 10 minutes before giving up.

II. Emergency Situations Where the Technique Applies

A. Heart disease
B. Seizures
C. Trauma
D. Lung disease
E. Heat stroke
F. Shock
G. Poisonings
H. Any other circumstances that cause the heart to stop

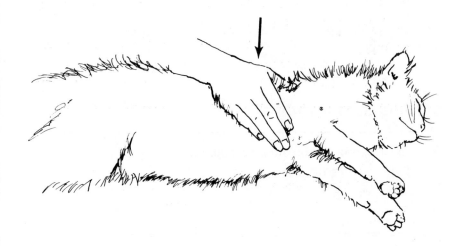

HOW TO MAKE A CAT MUZZLE

It may be necessary in certain cases to rely on a muzzle to help prevent a cat from biting when the cat is injured or extremely ill. A commercial muzzle (illustrated on page 46) is highly preferable to a homemade muzzle because it is easier to use and is often more effective. If a commercial muzzle is not available, however, a homemade muzzle is simple to construct.

NOTE: Never apply a muzzle if the cat is having difficulty breathing or is vomiting.

I. First-Aid Materials

A. Paper cup or styrofoam cup (approximately 8 ounces)
B. Two 6" strips of gauze
C. Adhesive tape
D. Scissors

II. Technique Instructions

A. Cut a 1-inch hole in the bottom of the cup. See illustration on page 45.
B. Tape or thread one piece of gauze through the drinking edge of the cup at the 3 o'clock position and one at the 9 o'clock position.
C. Place the cup over the cat's mouth, and tie the strings behind the pet's head.

III. Emergency Situations Where the Technique Applies

A. Trauma
B. Any situation where the cat is difficult to handle.
C. Never apply a muzzle if the cat is having difficulty breathing or is vomiting.

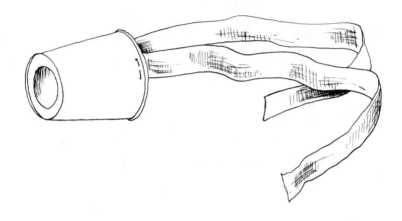

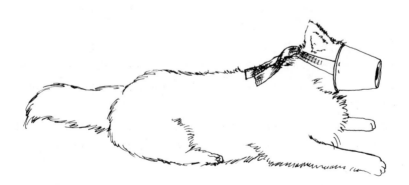

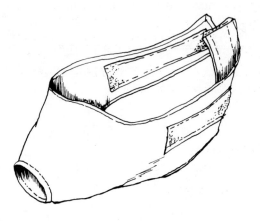

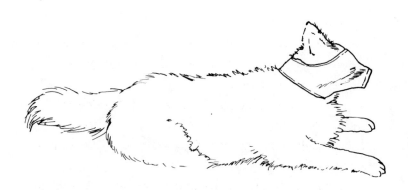

ELIZABETHAN COLLAR

An Elizabethan collar is a cone-shaped device that fits around the cat's neck. It is used to prevent a cat from instinctively licking or chewing an external injury. Because the cat's licking or chewing can cause additional damage and promote infection, the Elizabethan collar can help prevent serious complications.

I. First-Aid Materials

A. Medium-weight cardboard
B. Tape
C. Scissors
D. Or instead of the above items, a commercial Elizabethan collar

II. Technique Instructions

A. To construct a homemade Elizabethan collar, perform the following (as illustrated on page 49):
   (1) Draw a 6 to 8-inch diameter circle on the cardboard.
   (2) Cut out this circle.
   (3) Cut a circular hole the size of the cat's neck out of the center of the larger circle.
   (4) Make one cut from the outside diameter to the inside hole.
   (5) Slip the cardboard cut-out over the pet's head and secure the edges with tape to form a cone-like shape.
B. Fasten the collar securely, but make sure that it does not impede the cat's breathing. It should be loose enough for you to slip one finger under the collar. The collar should be long enough to keep the pet from licking and chewing. It may take the cat some

time to get used to the collar while walking, eating, and drinking.

C. Make sure the cat will eat and drink while wearing its collar.

III. Emergency Situations Where the Technique Applies

A. Skin irritations
B. Protruding organs
C. Bite wound abscess
D. Traumas
E. Other problems where the cat may make an injury worse by licking or chewing

---

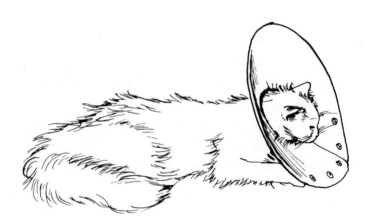

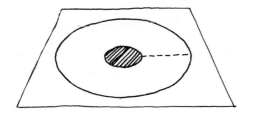

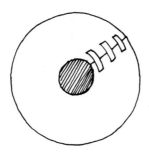

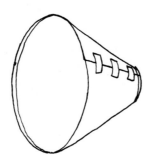

PART 3

—

HELP FOR THE PROBLEM

INTRODUCTORY
INFORMATION

Part 3 of this book is designed to provide a quick reference for treating many emergencies. Although this material does apply to a wide variety of emergencies, there are situations that may fall outside the scope of this book.

Part 3 of this book will enable you to find information in two ways: (1) by looking up the disease or condition, or (2) by looking up the primary symptom you observe. All information in both sections is in alphabetical order.

For simplicity, we use the term "symptom" to refer to both symptoms (things observed or experienced from the cat's point of view) and signs (things observed from the person's point of view). Note that for any given disease or condition, some or all of the symptoms listed may be present. Logically, the more symptoms you observe, the more likely you are to make a proper diagnosis. However, because there are many totally different diseases and conditions that have similar symptoms, it is important that you contact a veterinarian as soon as possible to ensure a proper diagnosis.

PROBLEM/CONDITION – ABRASIONS

I.   Symptoms (some or all may be present)

A.   Red skin
B.   Missing hair
C.   Painful area

II.   First-Aid Materials

A.   Contact-lens saline solution or water
B.   Antibacterial soap
C.   Clippers or scissors
D.   Antibiotic ointment (e.g., Polysporin®)
E.   Wrap material and/or Elizabethan collar

III.   First Aid

A.   Clip hair away from abrasion.
B.   Cleanse the abrasion using soap and saline solution or water.
C.   Apply antibiotic ointment to the abrasion.
D.   If necessary, apply a wrap over the abrasion and/or use an Elizabethan collar to keep the cat from licking, scratching or chewing the area. See page 35 on Wrapping a Wound and page 47 on how to make an Elizabethan collar.
E.   Seek veterinary help if the cat's discomfort persists.

PROBLEM/CONDITION – ABSCESS

The most common sites for bite wound abscesses are the legs, face, back and tail base. Bite wound abscesses on the leg are a more common cause of lameness in cats than are fractures. When a bite occurs, infection enters the puncture. The puncture then heals, and the infection festers under the skin resulting in a painful, swollen area filled with pus. This infection often spreads into the bloodstream causing serious illness.

I. Symptoms (some or all may be present)

A. The affected area is often swollen.

B. The area is often hot to the touch.

C. The cat may show other signs of illness like depression, lack of appetite, and fever.

D. There may be a healed puncture wound.

E. There may be a cloudy, bloody discharge present if the abscess breaks open.

F. If the abscess is on the leg, the cat may be lame.

II. First-Aid Materials

A. Warm compresses

B. Paper towels

54

III. First Aid

A. Locate wound. (Look for healed puncture wounds.)
B. Take pet's temperature.
C. Apply warm compresses to area to promote drainage of the abscess until a veterinarian can be contacted. The warm compresses may cause the abscess to rupture and spill out blood and pus. This will make the pet feel better because the infection is being removed from the body. Be prepared to clean up a mess.
D. Veterinary care is important; abscesses are generally treated with antibiotics, and some cats require sedation to promote better drainage of the infection.

PROBLEM/CONDITION – ACETAMINOPHEN (TYLENOL®) TOXICITY

Like many human drugs, Tylenol® is toxic to cats. In fact, one capsule may be lethal if the cat does not receive veterinary treatment. No medications of any kind should be given to a cat without instructions from a veterinarian. And because cats are curious by nature, all drugs should be kept out of your cat's reach to prevent accidental ingestion.

I.   Symptoms (some or all may be present)

A.   Listlessness
B.   Difficult breathing
C.   Vomiting and/or diarrhea
D.   Dark-colored urine

II.   First-Aid Materials

A.   Hydrogen peroxide
B.   Eyedropper

III.   First Aid

A.   If the cat is conscious, induce vomiting immediately by feeding the pet 1 teaspoon of hydrogen peroxide (mixed with 1 teaspoon milk if available). If the cat will not drink the mixture or if there is no milk available, then force-feed the cat the hydrogen peroxide using an eyedropper. If vomiting does not occur within 10 minutes, repeat the procedure up to two times.

B.   Contact a veterinarian for further treatment regardless of whether you are successful at inducing your cat to vomit.

PROBLEM/CONDITION –
ALLERGIES

Allergies in cats can be caused by a number of irritants. In people, allergies often cause sneezing, runny eyes, and wheezing, whereas in cats allergies usually cause itching and rashes.

Some skin irritations would not be considered life-threatening emergencies, but the degree of discomfort for the cat may be great. This section applies to both skin emergencies and minor skin irritations.

I. Symptoms (some or all may be present)

A. Red skin
B. Missing hair
C. Painful area
D. Cat scratching itself

II. First-Aid Materials

A. Moisturizing shampoo
B. Elizabethan collar

III. First Aid

A. If your cat will tolerate it, shampooing the pet will likely provide temporary relief from its symptoms. Use a shampoo for cats (moisturizing shampoo is best). While restraining the cat, lather the pet and let stand for 15-20 minutes. Rinse well. Consult your veterinarian for the proper type of shampoo and for specific instructions.

B. If the cat is biting itself, it may be necessary to apply an Elizabethan collar to prevent more damage to the skin. See page 47 on how to make and use an Elizabethan collar.

PROBLEM/CONDITION – ANEMIA

Anemia has many causes, but regardless of the origin of the anemia, the result is an inability of the blood to carry oxygen. It is important that the cat receive proper diagnosis of the condition from a veterinarian so that appropriate treatment can be administered.

I.   Symptoms (some or all may be present)

A.   Listlessness and depression
B.   Pale or white gums
C.   Loss of appetite
D.   Labored breathing
E.   Collapse

II.   First Aid

A.   The cat should see a veterinarian for proper diagnosis as soon as possible.
B.   Minimize stress during handling and transportation.
C.   Feed the cat a balanced cat-diet with an appropriate vitamin supplement prescribed by your veterinarian. Hand feed if necessary.

PROBLEM/CONDITION – ANTIFREEZE TOXICITY

Antifreeze is a common poison to pets for three reasons: it is a commonly-used product; it is often improperly discarded; and it is sweet to the taste.

Antifreeze contains ethylene glycol which, when metabolized, causes kidney damage that is usually fatal. Even a small amount will cause severe illness or death. Because the toxin is rapidly absorbed, symptoms may appear as early as one hour after ingestion. Symptoms are vague and mimic those of many other conditions and diseases.

I. Symptoms (some or all may be present)

A. Increased thirst
B. Vomiting and diarrhea
C. Depression
D. Loss of coordination
E. Kidney failure (sometimes preceded by apparent improvement in the cat's condition)

II. First-Aid Materials

A. Hydrogen peroxide
B. Liquor (e.g., vodka, whiskey, gin, rum)
C. Eyedropper

III. First Aid

A. If an exposure is suspected, induce vomiting by feeding the cat
   1 teaspoon of hydrogen peroxide (mixed with 1 teaspoon milk if
   available). If the cat will not drink the mixture or if there is no
   milk available, then force-feed the cat the hydrogen peroxide
   using an eyedropper. If vomiting does not occur within
   10 minutes, repeat the procedure up to two times.
B. Get immediate veterinary help.
C. If a veterinarian cannot be found, then when vomiting ceases or
   if vomiting cannot be induced, feed the cat using an eyedropper
   1 tablespoon of liquor (e.g., vodka, whiskey, gin, rum) mixed
   with 1 tablespoon of half and half cream. (If half and half
   cream is not available, then use milk or water.) Wait 10 minutes,
   and if there are no signs of depression or intoxication, administer
   another 1/2 tablespoon of liquor mixed with 1/2 tablespoon of
   half and half cream. (The ethanol in liquor competes with the
   ethylene glycol metabolism decreasing the amounts that may
   cause damage to the kidneys. It also promotes increased
   urination to allow faster excretion of the poison.)
D. Seek veterinary attention for further treatment.

PROBLEM/CONDITION – ASPIRIN TOXICITY

Pet owners have a tendency to medicate their pets according to how they would treat themselves if they were ill. Unfortunately, many human drugs are toxic to cats, including aspirin. No medications should be given to a cat without specific instructions from a veterinarian. Also, cats are curious, and any drugs should be kept out of their reach to prevent accidental ingestion.

I. Symptoms (some or all may be present)

A. Depression
B. Digestive upset
C. Fever
D. Rapid breathing
E. Seizures
F. Shock
G. Anemia, bleeding and liver problems caused by long-term low-dose exposure

II. First-Aid Materials

A. Hydrogen peroxide
B. Eyedropper

III. First Aid

A. If the pet is conscious, induce vomiting immediately by feeding the cat 1 teaspoon of hydrogen peroxide (mixed with 1 teaspoon milk if available). If the cat will not drink the mixture or if there is no milk available, then force-feed the cat the hydrogen peroxide using an eyedropper. If vomiting does not occur within 10 minutes, repeat the procedure up to two times.

B. Contact your veterinarian for further treatment regardless of whether you have been successful at inducing your cat to vomit.

PROBLEM/CONDITION – BEE STINGS

Bee stings are less common in cats than in humans because the cat's coat protects it from the stinger. When a cat is stung, it is usually stung on an exposed area like the nose or mouth. Fortunately, severe allergic reactions are less common in cats than in humans.

I. Symptoms (some or all may be present)

A. Cat scratching and rubbing the area of the sting
B. Swelling
C. Enlargement of the lips or nose (because most stings are to the face and mouth)
D. Difficulty breathing (though less common in cats than in people)

II. First-Aid Materials

A. Ice
B. Towel

III. First Aid

A. Apply ice wrapped in a towel over the swollen, painful areas.
B. Seek veterinary attention for medication.

PROBLEM/CONDITION – BITE WOUNDS

I. Symptoms (some or all may be present)

A. Red skin
B. Missing hair
C. Painful area
D. Bite/fang marks

II. First-Aid Materials

A. Contact-lens saline solution or water
B. Antibacterial soap
C. Clippers or scissors
D. Antibiotic ointment (e.g., Polysporin®)
E. Wrap material and/or Elizabethan collar

III. First Aid

A. Clip hair away from wound.
B. Cleanse the wound using soap and saline solution or water.
C. Apply antibiotic ointment to the wound.
D. If necessary, apply a wrap over the wound and/or use an Elizabethan collar to keep the cat from licking, scratching or chewing the area. See page 35 on Wrapping a Wound and page 47 on how to make an Elizabethan collar.
E. Seek veterinary help for antibiotic therapy.

PROBLEM/CONDITION – BLEEDING

External bleeding may result from an abrasion or laceration, trauma (e.g., gunshot wound, hit by car), bite wound abscess or compound fracture. Internal bleeding may result from trauma that does not cause a break in the skin, injury to a large muscle mass, a bone fracture, a tumor, toxicity from rat poisoning or injury of an internal organ. Whenever significant bleeding occurs, immediate action is required to prevent shock.

I. Symptoms (some or all may be present)

A. Blood coming from a wound
B. Blood accumulating under the skin, looking like a bruise
C. Blood in the cat's urine, feces or vomitus

II. First-Aid Materials

A. Clean towel
B. Gauze sponges
C. Nonstick adhesive tape
D. Nonstick bandages
E. Gauze wrap

III. First Aid

A. For internal bleeding:
   (1) Seek veterinary assistance immediately.
   (2) While awaiting veterinary assistance, keep the cat warm by placing a 2-liter soda bottle filled with warm water (not hot water) against the cat. Cover the cat with a towel or blanket.
   (3) Monitor the cat's vital signs (temperature, pulse and respirations) every 15 minutes and record the information. Try to keep the cat's temperature within the range of 100-102.5 degrees Fahrenheit. If the cat's temperature rises above 102.5 degrees Fahrenheit, remove the warm soda bottle. If the cat's temperature falls below 100 degrees, place an additional warm-water soda bottle against the cat, but make sure the water is not hot and make sure the bottle is against the cat and not on top of or underneath the cat.

B. For external bleeding:
   (1) Locate the source of bleeding.
   (2) Using a clean towel or gauze sponges, apply direct pressure to the wound for 5-10 minutes.
   (3) If the bleeding does not stop, apply a wrap as follows:
      a) Press nonstick bandage to wound.
      b) Secure nonstick bandage to wound by wrapping gauze around the leg or body. The gauze should be pulled snug but not tight. The wrap tightness should not restrict the cat's circulation or breathing.
      c) Secure the gauze by applying adhesive tape to the wrap.
      d) Monitor the pet for any evidence of swelling to the limb below the wrap. If swelling occurs, then the wrap is too tight and should be removed immediately. If the cat's breathing is hindered, also remove the wrap.
   (4) If the bleeding was difficult to stop, do not attempt to clean the wound or apply antibiotic ointment because the clot may be disrupted and severe hemorrhage may resume.
   (5) For future reference, note the amount of blood loss from the

68

injury. If the injury seems severe, treat the cat for shock as follows:

a) Keep the cat warm by placing a 2-liter soda bottle filled with warm water (not hot water) against the cat. Cover the cat with a towel or blanket.

b) Monitor the cat's vital signs (temperature, pulse and respirations) every 15 minutes and record the information. Try to keep the cat's temperature within the range of 100-102.5 degrees Fahrenheit. If the cat's temperature rises above 102.5 degrees Fahrenheit, remove the warm soda bottle. If the cat's temperature falls below 100 degrees, place an additional warm-water soda bottle against the cat, but make sure the water is not hot and make sure the bottle is against the cat and not on top of or underneath the cat.

(6) Call your veterinarian immediately. For best healing, lacerations should be repaired as soon as possible (ideally within one hour after the injury). As more time elapses, the wound becomes contaminated and may not be able to be closed.

PROBLEM/CONDITION – BURNS

      Many burns are not evident when they occur because the fur often conceals the injury to the skin. However, in some cases the fur will be burned away, and the injury will be readily evident. Burns can result from a variety of sources including chemicals, plants, heat, electricity and hot water. Burns should always be treated as soon as possible.

I.   Symptoms (some or all may be present)

A. If the fur is still present, the area of the burn may feel like a thickened area under the hair coat.

B. The burned area may feel hardened and may or may not be painful.

C. The pet may lick or scratch at the affected area.

D. If the burn is not recognized early, the fur and skin may start to peel away from the cat's body leaving a deep, weeping sore.

E. Signs of secondary complications include weakness (from dehydration), infections and depression.

II.   First-Aid Materials

A. Pet shampoo

B. Contact-lens saline solution

C. Antibiotic ointment (e.g., Polysporin®)

III. First Aid

A. **If the burn was caused by unknown chemicals,**
   (1) Bathe the cat immediately to remove any remaining chemicals. Use copious amounts of water. If available, use a pet shampoo (lather, let stand for 10 minutes, rinse).
   (2) Rinse the burned area in saline, and then cover the wound with antibiotic ointment. If the cat licks or scratches the area, cover the burn with a wrap. (See Wrapping a Wound on page 35.)
B. **If the burn was caused by an acid,**
   (1) Rinse the area with copious amounts of water.
   (2) Apply a paste of 1 part baking soda to 2 parts water to the affected areas.
C. **If the burn was caused by an alkali,**
   (1) Rinse the area with copious amounts of water.
   (2) Apply a solution of 1 part vinegar to 4 parts water.
D. **If the burn was caused by electricity,**
   (1) Cover the wound with antibiotic ointment. If the cat licks or scratches the area, cover the burn with a wrap. (See Wrapping a Wound on page 35.)
   (2) Seek veterinary assistance immediately because electric shock can cause dangerous arrhythmias (i.e., heart damage).
E. Because burns can have serious side effects like dehydration and secondary infections, it is important to get prompt medical care.

PROBLEM/CONDITION – CHOCOLATE TOXICITY

Chocolate contains a substance called theobromine which cannot be metabolized readily by cats. Even in small quantities, chocolate may be toxic to your cat.

I. Symptoms (some or all may be present)

A. Moderate to severe vomiting and diarrhea
B. Excitability and nervousness
C. Muscle tremors and/or seizures
D. Heart failure

II. First-Aid Materials

A. Hydrogen peroxide
B. Eyedropper

III. First Aid

A. Induce vomiting if the ingestion has occurred within the previous 6 hours. To induce vomiting, feed the cat 1 teaspoon of hydrogen peroxide (mixed with 1 teaspoon milk if available). If the cat will not drink the mixture or if there is no milk available, then force-feed the cat the hydrogen peroxide using an eyedropper. If vomiting does not occur in 10 minutes, repeat the procedure twice if needed.
B. See a veterinarian for further monitoring and supportive care.

PROBLEM/CONDITION –
CHOKING

It is not normal for a cat to choke on its food. When choking does occur in cats, it is frequently the result of something being lodged in the cat's mouth that has no business being there (i.e., something other than cat food). Therefore, choking can often be avoided by taking some common-sense precautions. See the section on Prevention starting on page 8 of this book.

I. Symptoms (some or all may be present)

A. Drooling
B. Pawing at mouth
C. Collapse
D. Labored breathing
E. Anxious behavior

II. First-Aid Materials

A. 1-inch roll of tape
B. Pencil with eraser

III. First Aid

A. Open the cat's mouth to see whether a foreign object is lodged in the cat's mouth or throat, but take care to prevent being bitten. If necessary, use a small roll of first-aid tape as a wedge to keep the cat's mouth open to allow better access and to protect you from the cat's teeth. (See illustration on page 75.)

B. If the cat's airway is not blocked, wait for veterinary assistance before attempting to remove any object; your efforts could do more harm than good. If the airway is blocked, use the eraser end of a pencil to try gently to dislodge the object.

C. If fluid is causing the choking, try wiping the fluid from the mouth using a tissue. You may need to hold the cat with its head lower than its chest for approximately 5 to 10 seconds in order for the fluid to drain. Repeat this process no more than two times.

D. If the pet becomes unconscious:

    (1) Observe for breathing by watching the cat's chest rise and fall.

    (2) **If the cat is breathing**, proceed to Step F; do not use CPR.

E. **If the cat is not breathing**, proceed as follows:

    (1) Establish an airway by removing any debris from the cat's mouth or by moving the tongue from the back of the throat. (See illustration page 41.) Check for breathing by watching the cat's chest rise and fall. If the cat is breathing, proceed to Step F. Do not use CPR.

    (2) If the cat is not breathing, lay the cat on its side (and throughout these procedures keep the cat on its side). Check for a pulse by placing a hand over the cat's chest just behind the shoulder blade (see page 43) to feel the heartbeat or by placing a hand in the groin area to feel the femoral pulse.

    (3) Cup your hand(s) over the cat's nose and mouth to form a seal. Deliver 1 breath into the pet every 2 seconds. If the seal is proper, you should observe the cat's chest rise and fall.

    (4) If after you have delivered 5 breaths the cat does not show signs of breathing on its own or signs of consciousness, and there is no heartbeat, then have a helper place a hand just behind the cat's shoulder blades (as illustrated on page 43),

and apply gentle but firm compressions downward (compressing 1/2 to 1 inch) at a rate of 1 compression every 2 seconds. If a helper is not available, alternate delivering 2 breaths then 10 compressions. **Do not do any compressions if there is a pulse, no matter how faint.**

(5) Check for a pulse and breathing every 2 minutes. If there is no pulse and breathing, continue for up to 10 minutes before giving up.

F. Sedation may be necessary to remove a foreign object; if your attempt at home is unsuccessful, seek immediate veterinary care.

G. Regardless of whether the object has been removed, have your cat checked by a veterinarian as soon as possible for lacerations in the mouth and throat.

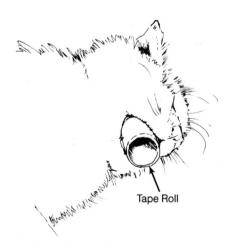
Tape Roll

PROBLEM/CONDITION – COLITIS

Colitis is inflammation of the colon. It has many different causes including allergic reactions, dietary indiscretions, foreign bodies, parasitic infestations and cancers. Even though not all causes of colitis are serious, the amount of discomfort the cat feels warrants the classification of colitis as an emergency.

I. Symptoms (some or all may be present)

A. Blood or mucous in the stool

B. Soft stools – If bowel movements cannot be observed, check under the cat's tail for stool pasted to the fur.

C. Foreign material (e.g., string, grass, etc.) protruding from the rectum – **Do not pull on these objects because they could tear or cut the bowels.**

D. Straining – (Note, however, that straining may be the result of a life-threatening urinary blockage. You should be able to see wet areas in the litter box from the cat's urination. See page 127.)

II. First Aid

A. If there is no foreign object protruding from the rectum and there are no signs of illness other than colitis, withhold food for 4 hours. (This time reference is for a normal, otherwise healthy, adult cat. Kittens and old cats should not be restricted from food for more than a couple of hours.) DO NOT withhold water from your cat. If your cat is not more comfortable within 4 hours or if other symptoms of illness are noted, such as lack of appetite, vomiting or listlessness, contact a veterinarian. Many times colitis requires treatment with antibiotics or anti-inflammatories.

B.   If any foreign object like grass or string is protruding from the rectum, do not pull on the object; it could lacerate the bowels. Instead, if the object is protruding more than two inches, cut the object with a scissors (to within 1 1/2 inches of the rectum) taking care not to cut the cat. Contact a veterinarian immediately.

C.   Add 1-2 teaspoons of bran flakes to your cat's meals to increase the fiber in your pet's diet.

D.   To aid your cat's digestion, feed your cat more frequently but in smaller portions.

PROBLEM/CONDITION – CONSTIPATION

I. Symptoms (some or all may be present)

A. Lack of stool in the litter box

B. Straining to go to the bathroom
   NOTE: Make sure the litter box has wet spots where the cat has been urinating. Straining from constipation could mimic a more serious problem like urinary blockage. Usually the straining associated with constipation will not appear as painful or as persistent as with urinary problems.

II. First-Aid Materials

A. Hairball preventive laxative

III. First Aid

A. Give your cat a laxative for hairballs as recommended by your veterinarian.

B. If the cat is uncomfortable or if more than 2 days have passed since a bowel movement, contact your veterinarian.

C. Most cats do not tolerate home enemas. An enema should be performed by a professional because a cat can be easily injured if it struggles during the process. If an enema is recommended by a veterinarian, make sure you never use a prepackaged phosphate enema because they are toxic to cats.

PROBLEM/CONDITION – DIARRHEA

The goal in helping a cat with diarrhea is to comfort the pet and lessen the symptoms until the cause can be determined. There are many causes of diarrhea including infections, dietary changes, foreign bodies, parasites and poisons.

I.   Symptoms (some or all may be present)

A.   Soft to watery stools
B.   Loss of appetite
C.   Painful abdomen

II.   First-Aid Materials

A.   Kaopectate®
B.   Eyedropper

III.   First Aid

A.   If there is no vomiting, feed the cat 1 teaspoon of Kaopectate® using an eyedropper.
B.   Withhold food for 2-4 hours if diarrhea is present and if there is no other symptom of illness. Withhold both food and water if the cat is also vomiting, but do not withhold water for more than 2 hours. Do not withhold water if the cat is not vomiting.

The time period for withholding food should be based on whether your pet is a normal, healthy adult versus a kitten, an elderly cat or a cat with any special or compromising conditions. (If your cat has diabetes or any other type of illness or medical condition, consult your veterinarian first before withholding food and water.) When you do resume feeding your cat, mix cat food (either canned or dry) with an equal amount of water, and make the serving size 1/4 the normal amount of cat food, but feed twice as often. Resume normal feeding within 1/2 to 1 day.

C. Note the frequency and substance of the diarrhea.

D. If symptoms persist for more than 4 hours, or if they worsen or return, contact the pet's doctor immediately.

PROBLEM/CONDITION – DIGESTIVE UPSET

The goal in helping a cat with digestive upset is to comfort the pet and lessen the symptoms until the cause can be determined. There are many causes of digestive upset, including infections, dietary changes, foreign bodies, parasites, and poisons.

I. Symptoms (some or all may be present)

A. Loss of appetite
B. Soft to watery stools
C. Painful abdomen
D. Vomiting

II. First-Aid Materials

A. Kaopectate®

III. First Aid

A. If there is no vomiting, feed the cat 1 teaspoon of Kaopectate® using an eyedropper.
B. Withhold food for 2-4 hours if diarrhea is present and if there is no other symptom of illness. Withhold both food and water if

81

the cat is also vomiting, but do not withhold water for more than 2 hours. The time period for withholding food should be based on whether your pet is a normal, healthy adult versus a kitten, an elderly cat or a cat with any special or compromising conditions. (If your cat has diabetes or any other type of illness or medical condition, consult your veterinarian first before withholding food and water.) When you do resume feeding your cat, mix cat food (either canned or dry) with an equal amount of water, and make the serving size 1/4 the normal amount of cat food, but feed twice as often. Resume normal feeding within 1/2 to 1 day.

C. Note the frequency and substance of the diarrhea and vomitus.

D. If symptoms persist for more than 4 hours, or if they worsen or return, contact the pet's doctor immediately.

PROBLEM/CONDITION – EYE EMERGENCIES

Examples of eye emergencies include corneal scratches, glaucoma, contusions, corneal ulcers, foreign debris in the eyes and popped-out (proptosed) eyes. A delay in treatment may result in permanent loss of vision.

I. Symptoms (some or all may be present)

A. Squinting
B. Excessive tearing (may be clear or cloudy)
C. Cat rubbing its eye(s) with its paw or rubbing its face on the ground
D. Enlarged eye(s)
E. Reddened white of the eye(s)

II. First-Aid Materials

A. Contact-lens saline solution

III. First Aid

A. If the irritation is minor, gently rinse the eye(s) with the contact-lens saline solution by applying several drops to the affected eye(s). This may dislodge any foreign debris causing the irritation. If the irritation is serious, contact professional help immediately.

B. If the symptoms persist, worsen or improve but then reappear, call the cat's veterinarian.

C. To keep the cat from further injuring the eye, apply an Elizabethan collar. (See page 47.)

D. Never apply human medicine to a pet's eye without the consent of a veterinarian.

PROBLEM/CONDITION – FRACTURES

The most common cause of fractures is trauma. Regardless of the cause, the single most important thing you can do to help the cat is RESTRICT ACTIVITY. By restricting activity immediately, you decrease the chances of the pet worsening the injury.

Many fractures are the result of severe trauma, such as getting hit by a car. An emergency involving a fracture should be treated with great urgency because the pet may have life-threatening internal injuries not immediately evident. If a fracture is compound (open to the air) or severely fragmented, the pet can hemorrhage and quickly go into shock.

I. Symptoms (some or all may be present)

A. Cats usually will not bear weight on a fractured leg.

B. Limbs may appear swollen.

C. Fractures are usually painful and do not improve with time.

D. Fractures of the ribs may be associated with difficult breathing.

II. First-Aid Materials

A. Gauze sponges and roll gauze

B. Tape

C. Muzzle

III. First Aid

A. If the cat is not having difficulty breathing and is not nauseous, then apply a muzzle to prevent the cat from biting.
B. Keep the cat still. If necessary, wrap the pet in a towel or blanket to restrict its movements.
C. Keep any open wounds covered with gauze and secure with tape.
D. If the open wound is bleeding profusely, apply pressure over that area.
E. Monitor the cat's vital signs (temperature, pulse and respirations).
F. Observe for other injuries.
G. Call your veterinarian for additional instructions.

IV. Transporting a Cat with Fractures or Back Injuries

A. Place a towel in the carrier.
B. Place a 2-liter soda bottle filled with warm water wrapped with a towel into the carrier.
C. If the cat is not having difficulty breathing and has not been vomiting, carefully place a muzzle on the cat prior to moving the animal. If at any time the cat has difficulty breathing or acts nauseous, remove the muzzle.
D. Avoid excess movement of the cat. Movement can be minimized by sliding the pet onto a small board or directly into a pet carrier.
E. To minimize discomfort, transport with the fractured side up.

PROBLEM/CONDITION – FROSTBITE

A cat's coat will not protect it from extreme cold. When temperatures or windchill fall below freezing, it is important that your cat has shelter. As with people, frostbite occurs when the extreme cold restricts blood flow to an appendage and thereby causes the tissue to die. The damage is frequently permanent. Frostbite may involve any appendage, but in cats most often it affects the tips of the ears. Exposure that causes frostbite can also cause death by freezing.

I. Symptoms (some or all may be present)

A. The ears or appendages may appear reddened and blistered. The symptoms may not be evident immediately after exposure to cold but will appear in a short period of time.
B. Frostbitten tissue will eventually turn dark and slough or scar.

II. First-Aid Materials

A. Contact-lens saline solution
B. Antibiotic ointment (e.g., Polysporin®)
C. 2-liter soda bottle

III. First Aid

A. If frostbite is suspected, immediately warm the ears or extremities in tepid water. Do not use hot water.

B.   If damage has already occurred, gently rinse the affected area in saline or water and apply antibiotic ointment.

C.   If the cat is chilled (hypothermic), fill a 2-liter soda bottle with warm water (not hot water), and place the bottle against the cat as illustrated on page 111. See page 95 for further information and instruction regarding hypothermia.

D.   Contact the cat's veterinarian for further instructions.

PROBLEM/CONDITION –
HEART DISEASE

Heart disease is a common occurrence in cats. The disease may be a result of a birth defect, infection, heart muscle disease, valve disease, or aging. Regardless of the cause, the condition may be very debilitating. Recognizing symptoms early and getting help as soon as possible will increase the cat's comfort level and improve the outcome.

I. Symptoms (some or all may be present)

A. Labored respirations (or gasping)
B. Weakness
C. Blue-tinged gums or tongue
D. Enlarged abdomen
E. Accelerated or depressed heart rate
F. Loss of consciousness

II. First-Aid Materials

A. Two 2-liter soda bottles
B. Blanket

III. First Aid

A. If the pet is unconscious and does not have a heartbeat or is not breathing, begin CPR immediately:
   (1) Lay the cat on its side (and throughout these procedures keep the cat on its side).

(2) Check for breathing by watching the cat's chest rise and fall.

(3) **If the cat is breathing,** proceed to Step B. Do not use CPR.

(4) **If the cat is not breathing,**

    a) Establish an airway by removing any debris from the cat's mouth or by moving the tongue from the back of the throat. (See illustration page 41.) Check for breathing by watching the cat's chest rise and fall. If the cat is breathing, proceed to Step B; do not use CPR.

    b) Check for a pulse by placing a hand over the cat's chest just behind the shoulder blade to feel the heartbeat or by placing a hand in the groin area to feel the femoral pulse.

(5) **If the cat still is not breathing,**

    a) Cup your hand(s) over the cat's nose and mouth to form a seal. Deliver 1 breath into the pet every 2 seconds. If the seal is proper, you should observe the cat's chest rise and fall.

    b) If after you have delivered 5 breaths the cat does not show signs of breathing on its own or signs of consciousness, and there is no heartbeat, then have a helper place a hand just behind the cat's shoulder blades (as illustrated on page 43), and apply gentle but firm compressions downward (compressing 1/2 to 1 inch) at a rate of 1 compression every 2 seconds. If a helper is not available, alternate delivering 2 breaths then 10 compressions. **Do not do any compressions if there is a pulse, no matter how faint.**

    c) Check for a pulse and breathing every 2 minutes. If there is no pulse and breathing, continue for up to 10 minutes before giving up.

B.   Keep the cat calm. Do not use excessive restraint or move the cat more than necessary.

C.   Keep the cat warm with the blanket and with the 2-liter soda bottles filled with warm water placed against the cat's body.

D.   Call your veterinarian.

PROBLEM/CONDITION – HEAT STROKE OR HYPERTHERMIA

Heat stroke is a common occurrence during the warmer months of the year. Cats are prone to overheating because they do not sweat. Other factors such as obesity, advanced age, infancy and poor ventilation also predispose cats to hyperthermia.

I. Symptoms (some or all may be present)

A. Panting
B. Weakness or collapse
C. Elevated temperature (from 105 to 110 degrees Fahrenheit)
D. Vomiting, diarrhea and/or lack of urine production
E. Seizures

II. First-Aid Materials

A. 2-liter soda bottle
B. Towel
C. Thermometer

III. First Aid

A. Take the cat's temperature.
B. If temperature is greater than 106 degrees, immerse the cat in

91

cold water.

C. Monitor the cat's temperature every 2 minutes to observe any change.

D. Stop the cooling process once the cat's temperature drops to 104 degrees. Do not wait until the temperature falls to normal because the cat's temperature may continue to drop.

E. If the temperature falls below 100 degrees Fahrenheit, keep the pet warm by covering it with a towel and by placing a 2-liter soda bottle filled with warm water (not hot water) against the cat.

F. Contact a veterinarian immediately to prevent shock and other complications.

PROBLEM/CONDITION – HIT BY CAR

In a situation involving serious trauma, such as being hit by a car, immediate care may be crucial to the eventual outcome. In addition to the damage caused by the physical impact, there is a high risk that the animal will go into shock. If your cat is not found by the road after being hit by a car, it may arrive home showing a varying degree of symptoms.

I.   Symptoms (some or all may be present)

A.   Weakness

B.   Lameness

C.   Difficulty breathing

D.   Bleeding

E.   Pale or purple gums

F.   Collapse

II.   First-Aid Materials

A.   Blanket and/or towels

B.   Gauze

C.   Tape

D.   Muzzle

E.   Contact-lens saline solution

F.   Antibiotic ointment (e.g., Polysporin®)

III. First Aid

A. Assess the danger to the pet (and to the caretaker if the injury has taken place near the road).

B. If the cat is having difficulty breathing, keep it upright and do not apply any unnecessary or overly-restrictive restraint.

C. If the cat is not having difficulty breathing and is not vomiting, then apply a muzzle to prevent the cat from biting.

D. Keep the cat warm by filling a 2-liter soda bottle with warm water (not hot water) and placing it against the cat. Cover the cat with a towel or blanket. This serves as both prevention and treatment for shock.

E. Transport the cat by placing it in a carrier, on a board or on a towel. If the cat has a fracture, to minimize discomfort, transport the cat with the fractured side up.

F. While awaiting veterinary care, wash and cover any open wounds.

G. For minor wounds, apply antibiotic ointment.

H. For additional information and instruction about specific injuries, see the appropriate section(s) of this book (e.g., fractures, bleeding, wound care, lacerations, wrapping a wound).

I. Get veterinary attention immediately.

PROBLEM/CONDITION – HYPOTHERMIA

Hypothermia (i.e., chilling) is a condition caused by exposure to cold. It may or may not be accompanied by frostbite. If your cat goes outdoors in cold weather, it is important that the pet has adequate shelter (e.g., a barn or a garage). Also note that your cat's general health, age, and build may make the pet more susceptible to hypothermia. Never let your cat outside if the temperature falls below 25 degrees Fahrenheit. Even in temperatures above freezing, your cat can become hypothermic if there is wind and rain. If left untreated, hypothermia can be fatal.

I. Symptoms (some or all may be present)

A. In early stages the cat may be shivering.
B. In later stages the cat will become stuporous, depressed, confused or even comatose.
C. The body temperature will fall below 99 degrees Fahrenheit.

II. First-Aid Materials

A. Thermometer
B. 2-liter soda bottles
C. Towels and/or blanket

III. First Aid

A. Take the cat's temperature.

B. If the temperature is below 98 degrees Fahrenheit, rewarm the cat carefully by placing a 2-liter soda bottle filled with warm water against the cat's body. (See illustration on page 111.)

C. Check the cat's temperature every 5-10 minutes. Keep the cat warm by keeping it covered with a blanket, even if its temperature returns to normal.

D. Because there is a danger of shock, immediately seek veterinary care.

PROBLEM/CONDITION – IBUPROFEN TOXICITY

Ibuprofen is an anti-inflammatory drug that, for cats, is even more toxic than aspirin. Because ibuprofen is a common household medication, cats often have easy access to the drug. Human medications should never be given to pets without the advice of a veterinarian.

I. Symptoms (some or all may be present)

A. Digestive upset
B. Bloody stool
C. Depression
D. Staggering
E. Increased thirst
F. Increased frequency of urination
G. Liver disease
H. Kidney disease
I. Seizures

II. First-Aid Materials

A. Hydrogen peroxide
B. Eyedropper

III. First Aid

A. If the pet is conscious, induce vomiting immediately by feeding the cat 1 teaspoon of hydrogen peroxide (mixed with 1 teaspoon milk if available). If the cat will not drink the mixture or if there is no milk available, then force-feed the cat the hydrogen peroxide using an eyedropper. If vomiting does not occur within 10 minutes, repeat the procedure twice.

B. Contact your veterinarian for further treatment regardless of whether you have been successful at inducing vomiting.

PROBLEM/CONDITION – INNER EAR OR VESTIBULAR DISEASE

The inner ear and vestibular system help control balance, posture and head position. Any injury, infection or inflammation in the ear can cause stroke-like symptoms. Early treatment is critical to prevent further damage and possible infection.

I. Symptoms (some or all may be present)

A. Tilted head
B. Disorientation/confusion
C. Stumbling and loss of coordination or balance
D. Walking in circles
E. Eyes involuntarily moving side to side

II. First Aid

A. Look in the ear to see if there is a discharge or something blocking the ear canal. If there is any debris in the ear, do not attempt to remove it; seek veterinary assistance to prevent further damage and infection.
B. If the cat is disoriented or appears to have a loss of balance or coordination, block off stairways and restrict the pet's activity. But make sure the cat has access to its litter box.
C. If the cat shows no sign of nausea, offer food and water by hand feeding; the cat's condition may prevent it from eating and drinking out of a bowl.
D. Seek veterinary care as soon as possible.

PROBLEM/CONDITION – INSECT INGESTION

Many varieties of insects can cause illness from ingestion. The symptoms will vary depending upon the type of insect, the quantity ingested, and the susceptibility of the particular cat. Because of the wide variety of insects, it is impossible to specifically identify which ones are toxic. In general, however, poisoning from insect ingestion is not a problem, and in particular, ingestion of an occasional fly, mosquito or lightning bug is typically harmless. There are some insects that have developed toxicity as part of their evolution to protect themselves from being eaten (e.g., the monarch butterfly), but these are the exceptions. Frequently with insect ingestion the risk of bites and stings in the cat's mouth is greater than the danger from ingestion.

I. Symptoms (some or all may be present)

A. Salivation from mouth irritation (from bites or stings)
B. Weakness
C. Vomiting
D. Diarrhea
E. Disorientation
F. Difficulty breathing
G. Seizures

II. First-Aid Materials

A. Hydrogen peroxide
B. Eyedropper

III. First Aid

A.   If it appears that the cat's mouth is irritated (e.g., if the cat is salivating or rubbing its mouth), flush the cat's mouth with fresh water using an eyedropper.

B.   If the pet shows any signs of illness from ingestion, immediately induce vomiting (unless the cat is unconscious or in a stupor) by feeding the cat 1 teaspoon of hydrogen peroxide (mixed with 1 teaspoon milk if available). If the cat will not drink the mixture or if there is no milk available, then force-feed the cat the hydrogen peroxide using an eyedropper. If vomiting does not occur within 10 minutes, repeat the procedure twice. Seek veterinary assistance for additional care.

C.   If possible, identify the type of insect.

PROBLEM/CONDITION – LUNG DISEASE AND RESPIRATORY DISTRESS

A cat suffering from respiratory distress does not receive enough oxygen to be comfortable or to function normally. This distress may be caused by many disease processes including infectious pneumonia, trauma, heart disease and cancer. Respiratory distress is life-threatening; contact a veterinarian immediately.

I. Symptoms (some or all may be present)

A. The cat may take short, shallow or rapid breaths or may pant.
B. The cat's gum or tongue color may be purple, blue, or pale.
C. The pet may be able only to sit upright with its elbows pointed outward; the cat may not be able to lie flat.
D. The cat may be depressed, but sometimes restless, due to the lack of oxygen.

II. First Aid

A. Avoid all stress. The least amount of stress may precipitate a crisis when the pet cannot breathe properly.
B. Do not monitor vital signs.
C. Plan the handling of the cat to minimize excitement. Never hold the cat tightly.
D. Keep the cat in an upright position (i.e., belly down). Never lay the cat on its back or side because those positions make breathing more difficult by putting extra pressure on the chest.
E. Contact a veterinarian immediately.

PROBLEM/CONDITION – PROTRUDING ORGANS

Various injuries and illnesses can result in the breakdown of vulnerable, weak areas of the cat's body. These areas include the eyes, abdomen and rectum. The things that most commonly protrude in a cat are a prolapsed rectum, a traumatic hernia with bowels exposed, and a popped-out eye. All of the above require immediate attention because these organs can dry out quickly causing permanent damage.

I. Symptoms (some or all may be present)

A. Most of these conditions can be recognized by observing the misplacement of the specific organ.

B. A prolapsed rectum may occur intermittently; the rectum may protrude only during times of straining, like during a bowel movement.

II. First-Aid Materials

A. Towel and/or gauze sponges
B. Contact-lens saline solution
C. Antibiotic ointment (e.g., Polysporin®)

III. First Aid

A. Contact a veterinarian immediately.
B. Soak a towel or gauze sponges with saline solution and apply to

any area of protrusion. This will keep the organs from becoming dehydrated and increase the chances of a better prognosis. Also, by covering the protrusion, you will help prevent the cat from mutilating itself. With a disembowelment in particular, cats will often chew on the exposed organs.

C. If the cat's eye is protruding, rinse the eye in saline every five minutes until a veterinarian can be reached. Do not apply pressure directly to the eye.

D. If the rectum is protruding, apply antibiotic ointment to help soothe the discomfort.

E. Use an Elizabethan collar if the cat is attempting to chew or scratch at the injury. See page 47.

PROBLEM/CONDITION – RAT POISON

Rat poisons are laced in a grain base that intrigues cats. When a cat eats rat poison, the poison interferes with the cat's ability to make vitamin K. Vitamin K is essential in causing blood to clot, and without the vitamin, a cat will hemorrhage internally. Because the symptoms from rat poison take several days to appear, early treatment is essential if an exposure is even suspected.

I. Symptoms (some or all may be present)

A. None for several days
B. Weakness – frequently the first symptom
C. Pale, white or bruised gums
D. Bruises on the cat's body
E. Bloody urine and/or stools
F. Blue-green feces or vomitus – some rat baits contain a blue-green dye
G. Death – may occur within 24 hours from the time symptoms develop

II. First-Aid Materials

A. Hydrogen peroxide
B. Eyedropper

III. First Aid

A. If exposure has occurred within 6 hours, immediately induce vomiting by feeding the cat 1 teaspoon of hydrogen peroxide (mixed with 1 teaspoon milk if available). If the cat will not drink the mixture or if there is no milk available, then force-feed the cat the hydrogen peroxide using an eyedropper. If vomiting does not occur within 10 minutes, repeat the procedure twice.

B. Regardless of whether you have been able to induce vomiting, seek veterinary care immediately. Your veterinarian will prescribe vitamin K as an antidote and may also prescribe medicines to slow absorption of the poison.

PROBLEM/CONDITION – SEIZURES

Seizures are common phenomena in cats. They can be caused by a number of problems, including blood sugar imbalances (sometimes from diabetes), head trauma, various poisons or a buildup of wastes in the cat's circulation (as a result of organ failure). Some seizures may be hereditary in nature.

Seizures are one of the most frightening events to watch. Try hard to stay calm so that you are best able to tend to your cat's needs.

I. Symptoms (some or all may be present)

A. Confusion prior to the onset
B. Lack of awareness of its surroundings, including unresponsiveness to the owner
C. Distressed meowing
D. Loss of bladder and/or bowel control
E. Twitching or convulsing
F. Collapse
G. After the seizure has ended, the cat may be confused, uncoordinated and possibly blind for minutes or even hours.

II. First Aid

A. Note the time on a clock to measure the duration of the seizure.
B. If the seizure lasts more than 2 minutes, get veterinary help

immediately; the condition may be life-threatening.

C. Move any objects that could cause the cat injury.

D. Block any stairways.

E. Never place your fingers in a cat's mouth during a seizure.

F. If the seizure stops and the cat appears lifeless, proceed as follows:

(1) Check for breathing by watching the cat's chest rise and fall.

(2) Establish an airway by removing any debris from the cat's mouth or by moving the tongue from the back of the throat. (See illustration page 41.) Check for breathing by watching the cat's chest rise and fall. **If the cat is breathing, proceed to Step G, and do not use CPR.**

(3) If the cat is still not breathing, lay the cat on its side (and throughout these procedures keep the cat on its side). Check for a pulse by placing a hand over the cat's chest just behind the shoulder blade (see page 43) to feel the heartbeat or by placing a hand in the groin area to feel the femoral pulse.

(4) **If the cat still is not breathing,**

    a) Cup your hand(s) over the cat's nose and mouth to form a seal. Deliver 1 breath into the pet every 2 seconds. If the seal is proper, you should observe the cat's chest rise and fall.

    b) If after you have delivered 5 breaths the cat does not show signs of breathing on its own or signs of consciousness, and there is no heartbeat, then have a helper place a hand just behind the cat's shoulder blades (as illustrated on page 43), and apply gentle but firm compressions downward (compressing 1/2 to 1 inch) at a rate of 1 compression every 2 seconds. If a helper is not available, alternate delivering 2 breaths then 10 compressions. **Do not do any compressions if there is a pulse, no matter how faint.**

    c) Check for a pulse and breathing every 2 minutes. If there is no pulse and breathing, continue for up to

10 minutes before giving up.

G. If the seizure stops at home, even if the pet seems normal, consult your veterinarian as soon as possible.

PROBLEM/CONDITION – SHOCK

Shock is an event that accompanies some diseases and injuries. It occurs when a series of compensatory mechanisms in the body goes awry. Problems that can cause shock include overwhelming infections, trauma (i.e., physical injury), severe vomiting and diarrhea, blood loss, and any other serious medical situation.

During the shock process, the body cannot keep up with the mixed signals that are being relayed. The body has a relative loss of blood due to changes in circulation or from bleeding. Changes in blood pressure shunt blood from vital organs like the heart, lungs, liver, kidneys and brain to other less important areas of the body. The result can be fatal if not treated early.

I. Symptoms (some or all may be present)

A. The cat may be depressed and/or disoriented.

B. The cat's vital signs may be decreased. Body temperature may fall, breathing may be shallow and pulse may be weak.

C. The cat's feet, tail, and ears may feel cold to the touch.

D. Note that immediately after an injury or other shock-inducing circumstance the symptoms of shock may be difficult to recognize, but they may develop quickly.

II. First-Aid Materials

A. 2-liter soda bottle

B. Blanket or towels

C. Thermometer

III. First Aid

A. Shock is a danger in virtually all medical emergencies. You should treat your cat for shock following any serious trauma regardless of whether you observe any symptoms.

B. Keep the cat warm by placing a 2-liter soda bottle filled with warm water (not hot water) against the cat. See illustration below. Cover the cat with a towel or blanket.

C. Monitor the cat's vital signs (temperature, pulse and respirations) every 15 minutes and record the information. Try to keep the cat's temperature within the range of 100-102.5 degrees Fahrenheit. If the cat's temperature rises above 102.5 degrees Fahrenheit, remove the warm soda bottle. If the cat's temperature falls below 100 degrees, place an additional warm-water soda bottle against the cat, but make sure the water is not hot and make sure the bottle is against the cat and not on top of or underneath the cat. See illustration on page 112.

D. Contact a veterinarian immediately so that anti-shock drugs, and possibly intravenous fluids, can be administered.

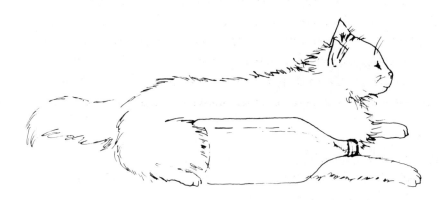

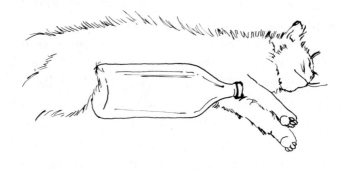

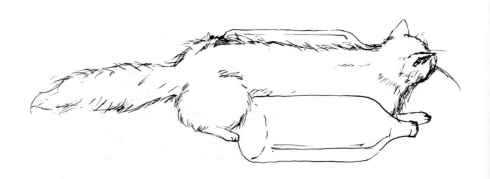

PROBLEM/CONDITION – SMOKE INHALATION

Smoke inhalation is often the cause of death when a cat is trapped in a fire. Smoke damages the respiratory tract thereby interfering with normal breathing; and, in addition, smoke contains the deadly gas carbon monoxide. It is important to note that the symptoms of smoke inhalation might not appear for as long as 1 to 2 days after the exposure.

I. Symptoms (some or all may be present)

A. Difficult breathing – short, shallow or rapid breaths, panting or coughing
B. Purple, blue or pale gums and tongue
C. Disorientation
D. Coma
E. Death

II. First Aid Materials

A. 2-liter soda bottle

III. First Aid

A. Move the cat away from the smoke.
B. Check for breathing. You should be able to see the cat's chest rise and fall.

C. If the cat is not breathing, establish an airway by removing any debris from the cat's mouth or by moving the tongue from the back of the throat. (See illustration page 41.) Check for breathing by watching the cat's chest rise and fall. **If the cat is breathing, proceed to Step E, and do not use CPR.**

D. **If the cat is not breathing,**

(1) Lay the cat on its side (and throughout Step D keep the cat on its side). Check for a pulse by placing a hand over the cat's chest just behind the shoulder blade (see page 43) to feel the heartbeat or by placing a hand in the groin area to feel the femoral pulse.

(2) Cup your hand(s) over the cat's nose and mouth to form a seal. Deliver 1 breath into the pet every 2 seconds. If the seal is proper, you should observe the cat's chest rise and fall.

(3) If after you have delivered 5 breaths the cat does not show signs of breathing on its own or signs of consciousness, and there is no heartbeat, then have a helper place a hand just behind the cat's shoulder blades (as illustrated on page 43), and apply gentle but firm compressions downward (compressing 1/2 to 1 inch) at a rate of 1 compression every 2 seconds. If a helper is not available, alternate delivering 2 breaths then 10 compressions. Do not do any compressions if there is a pulse, no matter how faint.

(4) Check for a pulse and breathing every 2 minutes. If there is no pulse and breathing, continue for up to 10 minutes before giving up.

E. Avoid all stress. The least amount of stress may precipitate a crisis when the cat is having difficulty breathing.

F. Do not monitor vital signs.

G. Plan the handling of the cat to minimize excitement. Never hold the cat tightly.

H. Other than when you are trying to resuscitate the pet, keep the cat in an upright position (i.e., belly down). Never lay the cat on its back or side because those positions make breathing more difficult by putting extra pressure on the chest.

114

I.   Fill a 2-liter soda bottle with warm (not hot) water and place it against the cat. See illustration on page 111.

J.   Contact a veterinarian immediately. It is easy to underestimate the severity of the cat's condition because some symptoms might not appear until 12 to 48 hours after smoke inhalation occurs.

PROBLEM/CONDITION – SNAIL BAIT

Snail bait is poisonous to pets because it contains the chemical metaldehyde. This product, like rat poison, is made with a tasty base that attracts not only snails but also cats.

I.   Symptoms (some or all may be present)

A.   Loss of coordination
B.   Muscle tremors or convulsions
C.   Increased heart rate

II.   First-Aid Materials

A.   Hydrogen peroxide
B.   Eyedropper

III.   First Aid

A.   Induce vomiting early if exposure is suspected. Do not attempt to induce vomiting if the pet is showing signs of poisoning (i.e., if it appears uncoordinated or is having muscle tremors or convulsions) because the pet could aspirate vomit into its lungs. To induce vomiting, feed the cat 1 teaspoon of hydrogen peroxide (mixed with 1 teaspoon milk if available). If the cat will not drink the mixture or if there is no milk available, then force-feed the cat the hydrogen peroxide using an eyedropper. If vomiting does not occur within 10 minutes, repeat the procedure twice.
B.   Contact a veterinarian immediately.

PROBLEM/CONDITION – SNAKE BITES

Bites from poisonous snakes pose a threat in many areas of the country. The severity of the bite will depend upon the type of snake, the age of the cat, the size of the cat, the number of bites, the location of the bites, and the amount of the venom injected.

I. Symptoms (some or all may be present)

A. Poisonous snake bites may appear as two punctures on the skin.
B. Nonpoisonous snake bites are usually shaped like a "U" because nonpoisonous snakes tend to have many teeth.
C. Poisonous snake bites tend to be especially painful.
D. The area around a poisonous snake bite will swell and may show bruising.
E. The cat may become depressed, paralyzed, comatose, and may die. These symptoms may be preceded by respiratory distress or by digestive upset.

II. First-Aid Materials

A. 2-liter soda bottle
B. Ice
C. Antibiotic ointment (e.g., Polysporin®)

III. First Aid

A. If you suspect that the bite is from a poisonous snake (see the symptoms listed above),
   (1) Wrap some ice in a cloth and place it against the wound. (The ice will slow the spread of venom.) Apply the wrapped ice over the swollen, painful area for 10 minutes. Wait 5 minutes, and then reapply for another 10 minutes.
   (2) Keep the cat warm by placing 2-liter soda bottles filled with warm water (not hot water) against the pet. (See illustrations on pages 111 and 112.)
   (3) Rush the cat to a veterinarian.
B. If the snake is identified as nonpoisonous,
   (1) Wash the bite wound with soap and water, and then apply antibiotic ointment.
   (2) Seek veterinary care for observation and antibiotic therapy because reptiles have many infectious bacteria in their mouths.

PROBLEM/CONDITION – SPIDER BITES, ANT BITES AND SCORPION STINGS

Several varieties of spiders, ants and scorpions can cause injury and illness in cats. The brown recluse spider and black widow spider are particularly venomous, though fortunately they are much less common than other spiders. Most ants are harmless in small numbers, but a colony of ants can pose a real risk. Scorpions are not native to much of the United States, but they (and tarantulas) are sometimes sold in pet stores.

It should be noted that some symptoms from spiders, ants and scorpions may not appear until 3 or 4 days after the bites or sting. These delayed symptoms may include paleness, blood in urine, fever, vomiting and shock.

I.   Symptoms (some or all may be present)

A.   Salivation, if bite or sting is in the cat's mouth

B.   Irritated area on skin

C.   Open sore on body

D.   Painful area

E.   Muscle pain

F.   Muscle contractions

G.   Fever

H.   Rapid or difficult breathing

I.   Paleness

J.   Vomiting

K.   Blood in urine

L.   Shock

M.   Paralysis

N.   Death

II. First-Aid Materials

A. Ice
B. Towel

III. First Aid

A. Seek veterinary care immediately.
B. Wrap some ice in a cloth and place it against the wound. (The ice will slow the spread of venom.) Apply the wrapped ice over the swollen, painful areas for 10 minutes. Wait 5 minutes, and then reapply for another 10 minutes.
C. If possible, identify the spider, ants or scorpion.

PROBLEM/CONDITION – STRYCHNINE POISONING

Strychnine is sometimes an ingredient in products sold to kill insects and rodents. The products are laced with a sweetener to attract the animal and generally contain enough strychnine that even ingestion of a small amount of the product will kill the pest. Unfortunately, strychnine is highly poisonous, and even a small amount will likely kill your cat. If your cat does ingest strychnine, immediate action is necessary.

I.   Symptoms (some or all may be present)

A.   Symptoms may appear within 2 hours of ingestion.
B.   The cat may appear to be apprehensive or nervous.
C.   Stiffness may develop, leading to severe seizures. These seizures can be provoked or exacerbated if an external stimulus occurs (e.g., a loud noise).
D.   Exhaustion and death may shortly follow the onset of symptoms.

II.   First-Aid Materials

A.   Hydrogen peroxide
B.   Eyedropper

III.   First Aid

A.   Induce vomiting if the pet is conscious and there has been a

121

suspected exposure. To induce vomiting, feed the cat 1 teaspoon of hydrogen peroxide (mixed with 1 teaspoon milk if available). If the cat will not drink the mixture or if there is no milk available, then force-feed the cat the hydrogen peroxide using an eyedropper. If vomiting does not occur within 10 minutes, repeat the procedure twice.

B. Keep your cat from injuring itself during any seizures by blocking off stairways and moving furnishings. If seizures do occur, follow the instructions on treatment for seizures, page 107.

C. Keep the cat in a calm, quiet environment.

D. Immediately seek veterinary help.

PROBLEM/CONDITION – TOAD POISONING

Many toads produce venom from glands in their skin. The amount of venom and its potency varies depending on the type of toad. The severity of symptoms you can expect your cat to exhibit from toad poisoning will depend upon the amount of exposure as well as the strength of the venom.

I. Symptoms (some or all may be present)

A. Salivation
B. Rubbing mouth
C. Shaking head
D. Dry heaves
E. Vomiting
F. Weakness
G. Difficulty breathing
H. Blue gums
I. Seizures
J. Collapse
K. Death

II. First-Aid Materials

A. Fresh water
B. Eyedropper

III. First Aid

A. Using an eyedropper, flush the cat's mouth with fresh water to remove excess venom.
B. If possible, identify the type of toad.
C. Seek veterinary care.

PROBLEM/CONDITION – TORN TOENAIL

With indoor cats it is important to keep their claws trimmed to prevent them from catching on carpets, draperies and furniture. If your cat does tear a toenail, it will be extremely painful for the pet, but the nail will eventually grow back.

I. Symptoms (some or all may be present)

A. Lameness
B. Nail hanging from paw
C. Blood coming from nail bed
D. Cat shaking its paw

II. First-Aid Materials

A. Muzzle
B. Gauze sponges
C. Gauze wrap
D. Tape
E. Nail trimmers

III. First Aid

A. Apply a muzzle if there is no evidence of difficulty breathing or nausea. (See page 44 if you need to make a homemade muzzle.)

B.   Do not attempt to remove a dangling claw. If the paw is bleeding, apply gentle but firm pressure to the paw to stop the bleeding.

C.   If the bleeding persists, wrap the foot with gauze wrap and tape. (See Wrapping a Wound on page 35.)

D.   See a veterinarian to have the nail trimmed or removed and for treatment to prevent infection.

E.   Keep the cat's healthy toenails trimmed to prevent injuries in the future.

PROBLEM/CONDITION – URINARY-TRACT IRRITATIONS

Urinary-tract problems are common in cats of all ages and breeds. These problems can quickly develop into emergencies because of the amount of distress the cats experience. In the worst case scenario, a cat may be unable to urinate because of a blockage; the poisons normally excreted in the urine accumulate in the cat's system causing severe illness which may include permanent organ damage, coma and death. If urinary-tract blockage is left untreated, death is imminent.

I. Symptoms (some or all may be present)

A. Urinating outside the litter box
B. Urinating more frequently
C. Straining while trying to urinate
D. Crying while urinating
E. Other generalized signs of illness (i.e., changes in behavior)

II. First-Aid Materials

A. 2-liter soda bottle
B. Clean litter box

III. First Aid

A. Observe the cat for urine output. The cat should be able to excrete small amounts of urine.

B. If no urine production is detected, the situation is urgent; the cat's urinary system may be blocked, and blockage is life-threatening. A veterinarian should be contacted immediately.

C. Monitor the cat's vital signs until a veterinarian can be reached.

D. Keep the cat warm by placing a 2-liter soda bottle filled with warm water (not hot water) against the cat.

E. Avoid lifting the cat around its abdomen to prevent discomfort and possible rupture of the bladder.

F. Even if urine is being produced, consult a veterinarian as soon as possible for diagnosis and treatment before the situation turns into a life-threatening blockage.

G. Do not encourage the cat to eat or drink because your veterinarian may determine that a urinary catheter is necessary, and insertion of the catheter may require a general anesthetic.

PROBLEM/CONDITION – UTERUS INFECTION

Infection of the uterus can occur for no apparent reason in a seemingly normal, healthy feline. The cause is generally hormonal, and prior to symptoms, there is no method of predicting when or whether it might occur. Infections of the uterus can be fatal. The unspayed, older adult female is at highest risk. When a cat's uterus becomes infected, it can fill with pus. Eventually the organ can burst, spilling infection into the abdomen, or the infection might be absorbed from the uterus into the bloodstream.

I. **Symptoms (some or all may be present)**

A. Increased thirst that precedes other signs
B. General signs of illness such as loss of appetite, vomiting, diarrhea or depression
C. A cloudy, foul-smelling discharge coming from the vulvar area under the tail
D. Tense and distended abdomen

II. **First-Aid Materials**

A. 2-liter soda bottle

III. **First Aid**

A. If any of these symptoms are noted, contact a veterinarian immediately. The cat may require an emergency spay before the uterus ruptures.

B. Do not lift the cat by putting extra pressure on the abdomen; lifting in that manner may cause the uterus to rupture.

C. To help prevent shock, place a 2-liter soda bottle filled with warm water (not hot water) next to the cat (as illustrated on page 111).

PROBLEM/CONDITION – VOMITING

The goal in helping a cat that is vomiting is to comfort the pet and lessen the symptoms until the cause can be determined. There are many causes of vomiting including dietary changes, infections, poisons, hairballs and obstruction from foreign objects that are undigestible. Sometimes vomiting is accompanied by diarrhea.

I. Symptoms (some or all may be present)

A. Loss of appetite
B. Salivation
C. Retching and/or vomiting
D. Painful abdomen

II. First Aid

A. If the cat is vomiting, withhold food and water for 2-4 hours. (But if your cat has diabetes or any other type of illness or medical condition, consult your veterinarian first before withholding food and water.) Do not withhold food and water from a kitten or elderly cat for more than 2 hours.
B. Note the frequency and substance of the vomiting. Is the food undigested or is the vomitus watery?
C. Note how long after a meal the vomiting occurred.
D. When you do resume feeding your cat, mix cat food (either canned or dry) with an equal amount of water, and make the serving size 1/4 the normal amount of cat food, but feed twice as often. Resume normal feeding within 1/2 to 1 day.
E. If symptoms persist, worsen or return within this 2-4 hour period, contact your veterinarian.

PROBLEM/CONDITION – YARD CHEMICALS

A variety of chemicals in fertilizers and pesticides can cause illness either from inhalation, contact or ingestion. Symptoms of illness may be delayed for days, but may be quite severe. Avoid exposing your cat to these toxins by keeping your cat indoors during and immediately after yard fertilization and spraying, and if you are using an insecticide indoors, keep your cat out of the room until the chemicals have dissipated. Never spray your cat with an insecticide that is not labeled specifically for use on cats.

I. Symptoms (some or all may be present)

A. Listlessness
B. Loss of appetite
C. Difficulty breathing
D. Vomiting
E. Diarrhea
F. Skin irritation from contact (typically the pads of the feet)

II. First Aid Materials

A. Shampoo

III. First Aid

A. If the cat gets chemicals on its fur, bathe the cat with cat shampoo (or any mild moisturizing shampoo if cat shampoo is not available). While restraining the cat, apply the shampoo and let it stand for 10 minutes before rinsing well.

B.   Seek veterinary assistance for additional advice and treatment.

SYMPTOM –
BLEEDING
(from abrasions and lacerations)

The most common problems that cause bleeding include abrasions and lacerations. When external bleeding does occur, you must get it under control as quickly as possible. An injury that causes significant blood loss may cause the cat to go into shock. (See Problem/Condition - Shock.)

I.   First-Aid Materials

A.   Clean towel
B.   Gauze sponges
C.   Nonstick adhesive tape
D.   Nonstick bandages
E.   Gauze wrap
F.   Antibiotic ointment (e.g., Polysporin®)

II.   First Aid

A.   Using a clean towel or sterile sponges, apply direct pressure to the area of bleeding for 5-10 minutes. If the bleeding does not stop, you may apply a wrap using the following procedure:
(1)   Press nonstick bandage to wound.
(2)   Secure nonstick bandage to wound by wrapping gauze around the cat's leg or body. The gauze should be pulled snug but not tight. The wrap should not restrict the cat's circulation or breathing.

(3) Secure the gauze by applying adhesive tape to the wrap.

(4) Monitor the pet for any evidence of swelling to the limb below the wrap. If swelling occurs, the wrap is too tight, and you should loosen it immediately. If the cat's breathing is hindered, also loosen or remove the wrap.

(5) Do not attempt to apply a tourniquet, even if the injury is a severed tail.

B. If the bleeding was difficult to stop, do not attempt to clean the wound or apply antibiotic ointment because the clot may be disrupted and severe hemorrhage may resume.

C. For future reference, note the amount of blood loss from the injury.

D. For serious lacerations, confine the cat to prevent activity.

E. For minor wounds, apply antibiotic ointment.

F. If the injury seems severe, treat the cat for shock as follows:

(1) Keep the cat warm by placing a 2-liter soda bottle filled with warm water (not hot water) against the cat. Cover the cat with a towel or blanket.

(2) Monitor the cat's vital signs (temperature, pulse and respirations) every 15 minutes and record the information. Try to keep the cat's temperature within the range of 100-102.5 degrees Fahrenheit. If the cat's temperature rises above 102.5 degrees Fahrenheit, remove the warm soda bottle. If the cat's temperature falls below 100 degrees, place an additional warm-water soda bottle against the cat, but make sure the water is not hot and make sure the bottle is against the cat and not on top of or underneath the cat.

G. Call your veterinarian immediately. For best healing, lacerations should be repaired as soon as possible (ideally within one hour after the injury). As more time elapses, the wound becomes contaminated and may not be able to be closed.

SYMPTOM – BLEEDING
(from bite wound abscesses)

Sometimes minor wounds can become infected, especially if the cause of the wound is a bite. With bite wounds, the skin may heal with an infection beneath it. The cat's immune system will attempt to isolate the infection, and the result can be the formation of a pocket of bacteria and pus called an abscess. The abscess may spread either inward through the bloodstream or outward through the skin. If the infection spreads inward, the resulting infection can damage internal organs. If it moves outward, it may rupture, and blood and pus will drain from the opening. The opening will appear as if something has eaten a hole in the animal, and it may be as large as a half-inch or more in diameter. The rupture and accompanying drainage may look frightening, but it is actually good for the cat because it helps get rid of the infection.

I.   First-Aid Materials

A.   Warm compresses
B.   Paper towels
C.   Antibiotic ointment (e.g., Polysporin®)

II.   First Aid

A.   Locate wound. (Look for healed puncture wounds.)
B.   Take pet's temperature.
C.   Apply warm compresses to area to promote drainage of the abscess until a veterinarian can be contacted. The warm

136

compresses may cause the abscess to rupture and spill out blood and pus. This will make the pet feel better because the infection is being removed from the body. Be prepared to clean up a mess.

D. Apply antibiotic ointment to the wound.
E. Contact a veterinarian. Your pet may need prescription antibiotics or may require sedation to promote better drainage of an infected wound.

SYMPTOM –
BLEEDING
(from gunshot wounds)

If your cat is ever a victim of a shooting, it may be critical that you get the bleeding under control as fast as possible. Also, you may need to treat the cat for shock. (See Problem/Condition - Shock.)

I. First-Aid Materials

A. Clean towel
B. Gauze sponges
C. Nonstick adhesive tape
D. Nonstick bandages
E. Gauze wrap

II. First Aid

A. Locate the source of bleeding.
B. DO NOT attempt to remove pellets or bullets.
C. Using a clean towel or sterile sponges, apply direct pressure to the area of bleeding for 5-10 minutes. If the bleeding does not stop, you may apply a wrap using the following procedure:
(1) Press nonstick bandage to wound.
(2) Secure nonstick bandage to wound by wrapping gauze around the cat's leg or body. The gauze should be pulled snug but not tight. The wrap should not restrict the cat's circulation or breathing.

(3) Secure the gauze by applying adhesive tape to the wrap.

(4) Monitor the pet for any evidence of swelling to the limb below the wrap. If swelling occurs, then the wrap is too tight, and you should loosen it immediately. If the cat's breathing is hindered, also loosen or remove the wrap.

D. For future reference, note the amount of blood loss from the injury.

E. If the bleeding was difficult to stop, do not attempt to clean the wound or apply antibiotic ointment because the clot may be disrupted and severe hemorrhage may resume.

F. Confine the cat to prevent activity.

G. Treat the cat for shock as follows:

(1) Keep the cat warm by placing a 2-liter soda bottle filled with warm water (not hot water) against the cat. Cover the cat with a towel or blanket.

(2) Monitor the cat's vital signs (temperature, pulse and respirations) every 15 minutes and record the information. Try to keep the cat's temperature within the range of 100-102.5 degrees Fahrenheit. If the cat's temperature rises above 102.5 degrees Fahrenheit, remove the warm soda bottle. If the cat's temperature falls below 100 degrees, place an additional warm-water soda bottle against the cat, but make sure the water is not hot and make sure the bottle is against the cat and not on top of or underneath the cat.

H. Call your veterinarian immediately.

SYMPTOM – BLEEDING
(from trauma, in general)

Often an emergency will involve some type of hemorrhage. The bleeding may be mild, moderate, or severe. Severe hemorrhage may involve the severing of an artery, injury to a large muscle mass, a fracture of a bone, toxicity due to rat poisoning, or internal trauma to an organ. If the blood pools quickly or pumps in spurts, you can assume it is serious. Immediate action is required to prevent shock.

Whenever there is serious trauma, there is a possibility of internal bleeding and shock. Seek veterinary assistance immediately.

I.   First-Aid Materials

A.   Clean towel
B.   Gauze sponges
C.   Nonstick adhesive tape
D.   Nonstick bandages
E.   Gauze wrap

II.   First Aid

A.   Locate the source of bleeding.
B.   Using a clean towel or gauze sponges, apply direct pressure to the wound for 5-10 minutes.
C.   A wrap may be applied to the wound if bleeding does not stop:
     (1) Press nonstick bandages to wound.

(2) Secure nonstick bandages to wound by wrapping gauze around the cat's leg or body. The gauze should be pulled snug but not tight. The wrap should not restrict the cat's circulation or breathing.

(3) Secure the gauze by applying adhesive tape to the wrap.

(4) Monitor the pet for any evidence of swelling to the limb below the wrap. If swelling occurs, then the wrap is too tight, and you should loosen it immediately. If the cat's breathing is hindered, also loosen or remove the wrap.

D. If the bleeding has stopped, do not attempt to clean the wound or apply antibiotic ointment because the clot may be disrupted and severe hemorrhage may resume.

E. For future reference, note the amount of blood loss from the injury.

F. Treat the cat for shock as follows:

(1) Keep the cat warm by placing a 2-liter soda bottle filled with warm water (not hot water) against the cat. Cover the cat with a towel or blanket.

(2) Monitor the cat's vital signs (temperature, pulse and respirations) every 15 minutes and record the information. Try to keep the cat's temperature within the range of 100-102.5 degrees Fahrenheit. If the cat's temperature rises above 102.5 degrees Fahrenheit, remove the warm soda bottle. If the cat's temperature falls below 100 degrees, place an additional warm-water soda bottle against the cat, but make sure the water is not hot and make sure the bottle is against the cat and not on top of or underneath the cat.

G. Lacerations are best repaired within a 1-hour time frame. As time elapses, the wound becomes contaminated and may not be able to be closed.

H. Trauma may be accompanied by internal bleeding. After any severe trauma, make sure your pet receives veterinary care to identify any problems you may be unable to detect.

SYMPTOM –
BREATHING DIFFICULTIES

I.   Problems/Conditions with that Symptom

A.   Heart disease
B.   Lung disease
C.   Heat stroke
D.   Internal bleeding
E.   Shock/trauma
F.   Anemia
G.   Fractured ribs
H.   Poisoning
I.   Asthma
J.   Obstruction of the airway
K.   Bee and scorpion stings
L.   Smoke inhalation
M.   Most other medical emergencies

II.   First-Aid Materials

A.   Two 2-liter soda bottles
B.   Blanket

III. First Aid

A.   Avoid all stress. The least bit of stress may precipitate a crisis
     when the pet cannot breathe.

B. Do not monitor vital signs.

C. Plan the handling of the cat to minimize excitement. Never hold tightly.

D. Never lay the cat on its back or side because this will compromise oxygen exchange by putting extra pressure on the chest.

E. Contact a veterinarian immediately.

SYMPTOM – BUMPS/LUMPS

I.   Problems/Conditions with that Symptom

A.   Allergy/hives
B.   Insect bites
C.   Drug reactions
D.   Bite wound abscess
E.   Tumor or cyst

II.   First-Aid Materials

A.   Towel(s)
B.   Ice

III.   First Aid

A.   If the cat is uncomfortable, place a towel moistened with cold water, or ice wrapped in a towel, over the irritated areas. This is especially soothing for hives and insect bites.
B.   Seek veterinary help. There are medications that may help give relief.

SYMPTOM –
CHOKING

I. Problems/Conditions with that Symptom

A. Foreign body
B. Aspiration of fluid
C. Hairballs
D. Nausea

II. First-Aid Materials

A. 1-inch roll of tape
B. Pencil with eraser

III. First Aid

A. Open the cat's mouth to see whether a foreign object is lodged in the cat's mouth or throat, but take care to prevent being bitten. If necessary, use a small roll of first-aid tape as a wedge to keep the cat's mouth open to allow better access and to protect you from the cat's teeth. (See illustration on page 75.)
B. If the cat's airway is not blocked, wait for veterinary assistance before attempting to remove any object; your efforts could do more harm than good. If the airway is blocked, use the eraser end of a pencil to try gently to dislodge the object.

C. If fluid is causing the choking, try wiping the fluid from the mouth using a tissue. You may need to hold the cat with its head lower than its chest for approximately 5 to 10 seconds in order for the fluid to drain. Repeat this process no more than two times.

D. If the pet becomes unconscious:

   (1) Observe for breathing by watching the cat's chest rise and fall.

   (2) **If the cat is breathing**, proceed to Step F; do not use CPR.

E. **If the cat is not breathing**, proceed as follows:

   (1) Establish an airway by removing any debris from the cat's mouth or by moving the tongue from the back of the throat. (See illustration page 41.) Check for breathing by watching the cat's chest rise and fall. If the cat is breathing, proceed to Step F. Do not use CPR.

   (2) If the cat is not breathing, lay the cat on its side (and throughout these procedures keep the cat on its side). Check for a pulse by placing a hand over the cat's chest just behind the shoulder blade (see page 43) to feel the heartbeat or by placing a hand in the groin area to feel the femoral pulse.

   (3) Cup your hand(s) over the cat's nose and mouth to form a seal. Deliver 1 breath into the pet every 2 seconds. If the seal is proper, you should observe the cat's chest rise and fall.

   (4) If after you have delivered 5 breaths the cat does not show signs of breathing on its own or signs of consciousness, and there is no heartbeat, then have a helper place a hand just behind the cat's shoulder blades (as illustrated on page 43), and apply gentle but firm compressions downward (compressing 1/2 to 1 inch) at a rate of 1 compression every 2 seconds. If a helper is not available, alternate delivering 2 breaths then 10 compressions. **Do not do any compressions if there is a pulse, no matter how faint.**

   (5) Check for a pulse and breathing every 2 minutes. If there is no pulse and breathing, continue for up to 10 minutes

before giving up.

F. Sedation may be necessary to remove a foreign object; if your attempt at home is unsuccessful, seek immediate veterinary care.

G. Regardless of whether the object has been removed, have your cat checked by a veterinarian as soon as possible for lacerations in the mouth and throat.

SYMPTOM – COLLAPSE

I. Problems/Conditions with that Symptom

A. Heart disease
B. Seizures
C. Lung disease
D. Heat stroke
E. Hypothermia
F. Internal bleeding
G. Shock/trauma
H. Infections
I. Poisonings
J. Urinary blockage
K. Anemia

II. First-Aid Materials

A. Two 2-liter soda bottles
B. Blanket

III. First Aid

A. If the cat appears lifeless, proceed as follows:
   (1) Check for breathing by watching the cat's chest rise and fall.

(2) Establish an airway by removing any debris from the cat's mouth or by moving the tongue from the back of the throat. (See illustration page 41.) Check for breathing by watching the cat's chest rise and fall. **If the cat is breathing, proceed to Step B, and do not use CPR.**

(3) If the cat is still not breathing, lay the cat on its side (and throughout these procedures keep the cat on its side). Check for a pulse by placing a hand over the cat's chest just behind the shoulder blade (see page 43) to feel the heartbeat or by placing a hand in the groin area to feel the femoral pulse.

(4) **If the cat still is not breathing**, perform CPR as follows:

    a) Cup your hand(s) over the cat's nose and mouth to form a seal. Deliver 1 breath into the pet every 2 seconds. If the seal is proper, you should observe the cat's chest rise and fall.

    b) If after you have delivered 5 breaths the cat does not show signs of breathing on its own or signs of consciousness, and there is no heartbeat, then have a helper place a hand just behind the cat's shoulder blades (as illustrated on page 43), and apply gentle but firm compressions downward (compressing 1/2 to 1 inch) at a rate of 1 compression every 2 seconds. If a helper is not available, alternate delivering 2 breaths then 10 compressions. **Do not do any compressions if there is a pulse, no matter how faint.**

    c) Check for a pulse and breathing every 2 minutes. If there is no pulse and breathing, continue for up to 10 minutes before giving up.

B. If the cat is conscious, proceed as follows:

(1) Keep the pet calm, and avoid unnecessary stress. Do not monitor vital signs, and do not use excessive restraint or cause excessive movement. Plan the handling of the cat to minimize stress. Never hold the cat tightly.

(2) Lay the cat upright (i.e., belly down). (If the cat is on its

back or side, there is extra pressure on the chest making it harder for the pet to breathe.)

C.   Seek immediate veterinary care.

SYMPTOM –
COUGHING

I. Problems/Conditions with that Symptom

A. Heart disease
B. Lung disease
C. Infections
D. Hairballs
E. Asthma
F. Smoke inhalation
G. Obstruction from a foreign object

II. First-Aid Materials

A. Cat hairball laxative/preventive

III. First Aid

A. If the cause of the cough is unknown, offer the pet 1 teaspoon of cat hairball laxative.
B. If the cough persists, see a veterinarian as soon as possible.
C. If the cat's breathing becomes labored, refer to Breathing Difficulties on page 142.

SYMPTOM –
DIARRHEA

I.   Problems/Conditions with that Symptom

A.   Heat stroke
B.   Shock/trauma
C.   Infections
D.   Poisonings
E.   Parasites
F.   Cancer
G.   Dietary changes or indiscretions

II.   First-Aid Materials

A.   Kaopectate®

III.   First Aid

A.   If there is no vomiting, feed the cat 1 teaspoon of Kaopectate® using an eyedropper.
B.   Withhold food for 2-4 hours if diarrhea is present and if there is no other symptom of illness. Withhold both food and water if the cat is also vomiting, but do not withhold water for more than 2 hours. Do not withhold water if the cat is not vomiting. The time period for withholding food should be based on

152

whether your pet is a normal, healthy adult versus a kitten, an elderly cat or a cat with any special or compromising conditions. (If your cat has diabetes or any other type of illness or medical condition, consult your veterinarian first before withholding food and water.) When you do resume feeding your cat, mix cat food (either canned or dry) with an equal amount of water, and make the serving size 1/4 the normal amount of cat food, but feed twice as often. Resume normal feeding within 1/2 to 1 day.

C. Note the frequency and substance of the diarrhea.
D. If symptoms persist for more than 4 hours, or if they worsen or return, contact the pet's doctor immediately.

SYMPTOM –
DISEMBOWELMENT

I.   Problems/Conditions with that Symptom

A.   Severe trauma
B.   Post-operative complications

II.   First-Aid Materials

A.   Towel and/or gauze sponges
B.   Contact-lens saline solution

III. First Aid

A.   Contact a veterinarian immediately.
B.   Soak a towel or gauze sponges with saline solution and apply it
     to the area of protrusion to keep the organs from becoming
     dehydrated.
C.   Keep the organs covered with the wet towel and/or wet sponges to
     keep the cat from mutilating itself. Cats will often chew on the
     bowels if they are exposed.
D.   Use an Elizabethan collar if the cat is attempting to chew or
     scratch the injury. See page 47.

SYMPTOM –
DROOLING

I. Problems/Conditions with that Symptom

A. Nausea
B. Gum irritation
C. Diseased teeth
D. Foreign body in mouth
E. Chemical or plant exposure
F. Contagious disease (e.g., rabies)

II. First-Aid Materials

A. Pet shampoo

III. First Aid

A. Determine whether your pet may have been exposed to a poison. If so, try to determine the type of poison. Then use the index of this book to find emergency treatment for ingestion of poison in general or, ideally, for ingestion of the particular substance.
B. If there was a flea chemical recently applied to the cat (i.e., that same day), bathe the cat with pet shampoo that does not contain flea chemicals to remove excess chemicals from the coat. Most drooling should stop within 30 minutes.

C. If poisoning or chemicals do not appear to be the cause, check the cat's mouth for diseased teeth, irritated gums and foreign objects by opening the cat's jaws and lifting the cat's lips. (See illustration on page 41.) Do not attempt to remove any object that is wedged in the cat's mouth unless the airway becomes completely blocked; instead seek veterinary assistance immediately.

D. If the cause is unknown and the drooling persists, withhold food and water temporarily and contact a veterinarian immediately.

SYMPTOM – EYES (RUNNY/SORE)

I. Problems/Conditions with that Symptom

A. Corneal scratches
B. Glaucoma
C. Contusions
D. Infections
E. Corneal ulcers
F. Foreign debris
G. Allergies

II. First-Aid Materials

A. Contact-lens saline solution

III. First Aid

A. Gently rinse the eye(s) with the contact-lens saline solution by applying several drops to the affected eye. This may dislodge any foreign debris.
B. If the symptoms improve but reappear, stay the same or worsen, call the cat's veterinarian.
C. If the cat is rubbing its eye, use an Elizabethan collar to prevent the behavior. See page 47.
D. Never apply human medicine to a pet's eye unless instructed by a veterinarian.

SYMPTOM –
HEAD TILT

The most common cause of a cat having its head tilted is an inner ear problem. Both the underlying condition and the head tilt often result in disorientation, loss of balance and coordination, and sometimes an inability to self-feed.

I.   Problems/Conditions with that Symptom

A.   Inner ear infections and swelling
B.   Trauma
C.   Cancers/tumors
D.   Foreign body in ear

II.   First Aid

A.   Look in the ear to see if there is a discharge or something blocking the ear canal. If there is any debris in the ear, do not attempt to remove it; seek veterinary assistance to prevent further damage and infection.
B.   If the cat is disoriented or appears to have a loss of balance or coordination, block off stairways and restrict the pet's activity. But make sure the cat has access to its litter box.
C.   If the cat shows no sign of nausea, offer food and water by hand feeding; the cat's condition may prevent it from eating and drinking out of a bowl.
D.   Seek veterinary care as soon as possible.

SYMPTOM – LAMENESS

I. Problems/Conditions with that Symptom

A. Fractures
B. Sprains
C. Bite wound abscesses
D. Bruises
E. Foot-pad injury (e.g., splinter, puncture, laceration)

II. First-Aid Materials

A. Gauze sponges and roll gauze
B. Tape
C. Tweezers
D. Antibiotic ointment (e.g., Polysporin®)

III. First Aid

A. Keep the cat still.
B. If lameness is caused by a splinter or similar foreign object, use tweezers to remove the object. Apply antibiotic ointment.
C. For any minor wound where bleeding control is not a problem, apply antibiotic ointment and keep the wound covered with gauze and secure with tape.
D. If the cat has a wound that is bleeding, apply pressure. (For

additional information, see Bleeding From Abrasions and Lacerations on page 134.)

E. Monitor the cat's vital signs (temperature, pulse, and respirations).

F. Observe for other injuries.

G. Call a veterinarian for additional instructions.

SYMPTOM –
LITTER BOX/BROKEN
HABITS

I.   Problems/Conditions with that Symptom

A.   Urinary-tract irritation
B.   Urinary blockage

II.   First-Aid Materials

A.   2-liter soda bottle
B.   Clean litter box

III.   First Aid

A.   Observe the cat for urine output. The cat should be able to excrete small amounts of urine. If no urine production is detected, it is a life-threatening emergency because the cat may be blocked and unable to urinate.
B.   If you suspect urinary blockage, proceed as follows:
  (1) Contact a veterinarian immediately.
  (2) Avoid lifting the cat around its abdomen to prevent discomfort and possible rupture of the bladder.
  (3) Keep the cat warm by placing a 2-liter soda bottle filled with

warm water (not hot water) against the cat.

(4) Do not encourage the cat to eat or drink because your veterinarian may determine that a urinary catheter is necessary, and insertion of the catheter may require a general anesthetic.

C. Other signs of a urinary tract problem include straining, frequent attempted urination and crying during urination. Even if urine is being produced, if you suspect that there is a urinary tract problem, consult a veterinarian as soon as possible for diagnosis and treatment before the situation turns into a life-threatening block.

SYMPTOM –
LOSS OF COORDINATION/
LOSS OF BALANCE

Loss of coordination or balance may result from a variety of causes, but one of the most common is an inner ear problem. The inner ear controls balance, posture and head position. If your cat's symptoms are accompanied by a head tilt, then whatever the underlying cause, it is possible there is a problem with the inner ear.

I.   Problems/Conditions with that Symptom

A.   Inner ear infections and swelling
B.   Trauma
C.   Cancers/tumors
D.   Foreign object in ear
E.   Poisoning or extreme illness

II.   First Aid

A.   Look in the ear to see if there is a discharge or something blocking the ear canal. If there is any debris in the ear, do not attempt to remove it; seek veterinary assistance immediately to prevent further damage and infection.
B.   Block off stairways and restrict the pet's activity, but make sure the cat has access to its litter box.
C.   If the cat shows no sign of nausea, offer food and water by hand feeding; the cat's condition may prevent it from eating and drinking out of a bowl.
D.   Seek veterinary care as soon as possible.

SYMPTOM – PROTRUDING EYE

I. Problems/Conditions with that Symptom

A. Trauma
B. Glaucoma

II. First-Aid Materials

A. Gauze sponges
B. Contact-lens saline solution

III. First Aid

A. Contact a veterinarian immediately.
B. Soak gauze sponge with saline solution and apply to the eye or apply several drops of saline directly onto the affected eye every 5 minutes. This will keep the eye from becoming dehydrated.
C. Do not apply pressure to the eye to stop bleeding.
D. Use an Elizabethan collar if the cat is attempting to scratch at the injury. See page 47.

SYMPTOM – PROTRUDING RECTUM

I.   Problems/Conditions with that Symptom

A.   Diarrhea
B.   Straining
C.   Colitis
D.   Foreign body

II.   First-Aid Materials

A.   Towel and/or gauze sponges
B.   Contact-lens saline solution
C.   Antibiotic ointment (e.g., Polysporin®)

III.   First Aid

A.   Contact a veterinarian immediately.
B.   Soak a towel or gauze sponges with saline solution and place on the rectum or apply several drops of saline directly onto the rectum to prevent the organ from becoming dehydrated.
C.   Apply antibiotic ointment to help soothe the discomfort and prevent infection.
D.   An Elizabethan collar may be utilized if the cat is attempting to scratch or chew at the injury. See page 47.

SYMPTOM – SCRATCHING SKIN/ IRRITATED SKIN

I. Problems/Conditions with that Symptom

A. Contact with plant resins

B. Frostbite

C. Burns

D. Abrasions

E. Bites and stings (e.g., insects, spiders, snakes)

F. Allergies

G. Fleas, lice and/or mites

H. Drug reactions

II. First-Aid Materials

A. Cat moisturizing shampoo

B. Elizabethan collar

III. First Aid

A. If your cat will tolerate it, shampooing the pet will likely provide temporary relief from its symptoms. Use a shampoo for cats if available, otherwise use any mild moisturizing shampoo. While restraining the cat, lather the pet and let stand for 15-20 minutes.

Rinse well. Consult your veterinarian for the proper type of shampoo and for specific instructions.

B.   If the cat is biting itself, it may be necessary to apply an Elizabethan collar to prevent more damage to the skin. See page 47 on how to make and use an Elizabethan collar.

SYMPTOM –
SHAKING HEAD/
SCRATCHING EARS

I. Problems/Conditions with that Symptom

A. Ear infection
B. Ear mites
C. Trauma (physical injury)
D. Bite wound abscess
E. Ear hematoma (swelling)
F. Toad poisoning

II. First-Aid Materials

A. Gauze sponges or cotton balls

III. First Aid

A. If there is debris in the ear flap, gently remove it by using a dry cotton ball or gauze sponge, being careful not to pack the debris into the ear canal. Do not use water or hydrogen peroxide because the moisture will promote infection.
B. Consult your veterinarian as soon as possible.

SYMPTOM – STRAINING

I. Problems/Conditions with that Symptom

A. Urinary tract irritation
B. Urinary blockage
C. Constipation
D. Colitis
E. Difficult delivery

II. First-Aid Materials

A. 2-liter soda bottle
B. Clean litter box

III. First Aid

A. Observe the cat for urine output. The cat should be able to excrete small amounts of urine. If no urine production is detected, it is a life-threatening emergency because the cat may be blocked and unable to urinate.

B. If you suspect urinary blockage proceed as follows:
   (1) Contact a veterinarian immediately.
   (2) Avoid lifting the cat around its abdomen to prevent discomfort and possible rupture of the bladder.

169

(3) Keep the cat warm by placing a 2-liter soda bottle filled with warm water (not hot water) against the cat.

(4) Do not encourage the cat to eat or drink because your veterinarian may determine that a urinary catheter is necessary, and insertion of the catheter may require a general anesthetic.

C. Other signs of a urinary tract problem include frequent attempted urination and crying during urination. Even if urine is being produced, if you suspect that there is a urinary tract problem, consult a veterinarian as soon as possible for diagnosis and treatment before the situation turns into a life-threatening block.

D. If a urinary tract irritation and blockage can be ruled out, see the sections on constipation (page 78) and difficult deliveries (page 282).

SYMPTOM – VOMITING

I. Problems/Conditions with that Symptom

A. Infections
B. Dietary change
C. Poisonings
D. Heat stroke
E. Shock
F. Foreign objects
G. Hairballs

II. First Aid

A. If the cat is vomiting, withhold food and water for 2-4 hours. (But if your cat has diabetes or any other type of illness or medical condition, consult your veterinarian first before withholding food and water.) Do not withhold food and water from a kitten or elderly cat for more than 2 hours.

B. Note the frequency and substance of the vomiting. Is the food undigested or is the vomitus watery?

C. Note how long after a meal the vomiting occurred.

D. When you do resume feeding your cat, mix cat food (either canned or dry) with an equal amount of water, and make the serving size 1/4 the normal amount of cat food, but feed twice as often. Resume normal feeding within 1/2 to 1 day.

E. If symptoms persist, worsen or return within this 2-4 hour period, contact your veterinarian.

SYMPTOM – WEAKNESS/DEPRESSION

Weakness and depression are vague symptoms associated with many diseases and conditions. Recognizing the symptoms is easy, but pinpointing the cause is difficult. Weakness and depression are often early symptoms of a more serious problem.

I. Problems/Conditions with that Symptom

A. Heart disease
B. Lung disease
C. Heat stroke
D. Internal bleeding
E. Shock
F. Trauma (physical injury)
G. Anemia
H. Fractured ribs
I. Poisoning
J. Asthma
K. Dehydration

II. First-Aid Materials

A. Two 2-liter soda bottles
B. Blanket
C. Thermometer

III. First Aid

A. Keep the cat calm. Do not use excessive restraint or cause excessive movement.
B. Monitor the cat's vital signs (temperature, pulse, respirations).
C. Keep the cat warm with a blanket and with the 2-liter soda bottles filled with warm water placed close to the cat's body.
D. Call your veterinarian.

PART 4

POISON BASICS

GENERAL PROCEDURES

Because some poisons are sweet to the taste and because of the inherent curiosity of most cats, poisons pose a substantial risk to your pet. Early recognition is critical to prevent complications or death.

I. Information About the Cat

A. Be ready to provide the following information to your veterinarian: owner's name, address and phone number and the cat's breed, age, sex and weight.
B. If you have more than one pet, note whether the others are affected.
C. Be able to describe the symptoms the cat is experiencing.

II. Information About the Exposure

A. Note the suspected substance.
B. Identify the substance ingested. Save the label or container of the suspected agent, if applicable. If the agent is a plant and cannot be identified, obtain a sample of the plant.
C. Note the time of exposure.
D. Note the amount of the substance ingested.

III. Steps to Get Help

A. Immediately contact the cat's veterinarian to see if treatment is necessary.

B. If you cannot reach a veterinarian, call the National Animal Poison Control Center for information (for a fee of $20 for five minutes at the time of this printing: 1-900-680-0000) or a local poison control hotline.

C. Follow the veterinarian's or the Center's recommendations.

D. If you need to induce vomiting, see page 39.

E. Observe for symptoms (vomiting, diarrhea, loss of coordination, lethargy, etc.). Symptoms may not be evident immediately.

LIST OF COMMON POISONS

I. List of Common Poisons (see note at bottom of list)

Acetaminophen*	Acids*
Adhesives	Alkalis*
Amphetamines	Antidandruff shampoos
Antidepressants	Antifreeze*
Antihistamines	Antipsychotics
Arsenic*	Aspirin*
Atropine	Barbiturates
Benzodiazepines	Bleach
Borates	Bromethalin
Camphor	Carbon monoxide
Chlorinated hydrocarbons	Chocolate*
Cholecalciferol	Coal tar
Cocaine	Creosote
Cyanide	DEET
Detergents	Drain cleaners
Ethanol	Ethylene glycol*
5-fluorouracil	Flea products*
4-animopyridine	Glue
Ibuprofen*	Insulin
Isopropanol	Ivermectin
Lead*	Limonene
Mercury	Metaldehyde
Methanol	Methylxanthines
Naphthaline	Narcotic analgesics
PCP	Petroleum distillates*
Phenols	Phenylpropanolamine
Pine oil	Propranolol

Pyrethrins   Rat poison*
Snail bait*   Strychnine*
1080   Terbutaline
THC   2,4-D
Xanthines   Zinc oxide

*See Part 6 starting on page 233 for more details.

NOTE: The above list does not include all poisons. Some substances that are not harmful to people are poisonous to cats. Many common household products contain chemicals that are poisonous to cats. It is reasonable to assume that anything that is poisonous to people is likely poisonous to cats. For plant poisons, see Part 5 of this book starting on page 181.

PART 5

—

POISONOUS PLANTS

INTRODUCTION TO POISONOUS PLANTS

Because of their small size and their unique metabolism, cats tend to be highly sensitive to poisonous plants. Many toxic substances require quick home treatment followed by immediate veterinary care. Veterinary follow-up is critical to prevent secondary effects of the poisons. Also, a veterinarian can monitor the cat for complications.

It is important to note that because of the huge number of plants in existence, this section of this book cannot possibly address every plant that is or may be toxic to cats. Also, some plants that are generally considered to be nontoxic may cause severe symptoms in a cat with an allergy to the plant. And some plants that are not toxic are sprayed with chemicals that may be poisonous. Therefore, you should be concerned whenever your cat eats any type of plant, and you should contact your veterinarian immediately.

ALOCASIA

I.   Toxic Portion of Plant

    A.   All parts

II. Symptoms (one or both may be present)

    A.   Digestive upset

    B.   Burning sensation in mouth

III. First Aid

    A.   Feed milk to your cat.

    B.   Call your veterinarian immediately.

    C.   Observe for symptoms.

ALOE VERA

I.   Toxic Portion of Plant

    A.   All parts

II. Symptoms (one or both may be present)

    A.   Diarrhea

    B.   Urine may turn red in color

III. First Aid

    A.   If your cat is alert, induce vomiting.

    B.   Call your veterinarian immediately.

    C.   Observe for symptoms.

AMARYLLIS (Hippeastrum)

I.   Toxic Portion of Plant

    A.   Bulb is most toxic.

II. Symptoms (some or all may be present)

    A.   Digestive upset

    B.   Excitement followed by depression, then coma

    C.   Possible death

III. First Aid

    A.   If your cat is alert, induce vomiting.

B. Call your veterinarian immediately.

C. Observe for symptoms.

APPLE (Malus)

I. Toxic Portion of Plant

    A. Leaves and stems contain cyanide.

    B. Dried, withering leaves are most toxic.

II. Symptoms (some or all may be present)

    A. Rapid breathing

    B. Dilated pupils

    C. Red gums

    D. Shock

III. First Aid

    A. If your cat is alert, induce vomiting.

    B. Call your veterinarian immediately.

    C. Observe for symptoms.

AUTUMN CROCUS (Colchicum)

I. Toxic Portion of Plant

    A. Mostly bulbs

II. Symptoms (some or all may be present)

    A. Oral irritation

    B. Digestive upset

    C. Kidney failure

    D. Excitement followed by depression, then coma – may begin approximately 8 hours after ingestion

    E. Shock with possible death – following initial onset of other symptoms

III. First Aid

    A. If your cat is alert, induce vomiting.

    B. Call your veterinarian immediately.

    C. Observe for symptoms.

AZALEA (Rhododendron)

I. **Toxic Portion of Plant**

    A.   All parts

II. **Symptoms (some or all may be present)**

    A.   Digestive upset

    B.   Heart failure

    C.   Depression

    D.   Drooling

    E.   Weakness

    F.   Coma

III. **First Aid**

    A.   If your cat is alert, induce vomiting.

    B.   Call your veterinarian immediately.

    C.   Observe for symptoms.

BIRD-OF-PARADISE (Strelitzia reginae)

I. **Toxic Portion of Plant**

    A.   Seed pod

II. **Symptoms (one or both may be present)**

    A.   Digestive upset

    B.   Disoriented walking (occurs within 30 minutes)

III. **First Aid**

    A.   Induce vomiting if ingestion was within 1 hour and your cat is alert.

    B.   If ingestion of plant occurred more that 60 minutes prior, feed milk to the cat.

    C.   Call your veterinarian immediately.

    D.   Observe for symptoms.

BLACK LOCUST (Rubinia pseudoacacia)

I. **Toxic Portion of Plant**

    A.   Bark

    B.   Green growth

    C.   Seeds

II.   **Symptoms (some or all may be present)**

    A.   Digestive upset

    B.   Heart failure

    C.   Depression

III.   **First Aid**

    A.   If your cat is alert, induce vomiting.

    B.   Call your veterinarian immediately.

    C.   Observe for symptoms.

BLEEDING-HEART (Dicentra)

I.   **Toxic Portion of Plant**

    A.   Top growth

    B.   Corms

II.   **Symptoms (some or all may be present)**

    A.   Digestive upset

    B.   Irritation of mouth with possible swelling of the throat

    C.   Possible asphyxiation

    D.   Central nervous system signs - tremors, seizures, staggering, loss of coordination, etc.

    E.   Possible death

III.   **First Aid**

    A.   If your cat is alert, induce vomiting.

    B.   Call your veterinarian immediately.

    C.   Observe for symptoms.

BOXWOOD (Buxus)

I.   **Toxic Portion of Plant**

    A.   All parts

II.   **Symptoms (some or all may be present)**

    A.   Digestive upset

    B.   Excitement or depression

186

C. Heart failure

III. First Aid

A. If your cat is alert, induce vomiting.

B. Call your veterinarian immediately.

C. Observe for symptoms.

BROAD BEAN (Vicia faba)

See Fava Bean on page 201

BUCKEYE (Aesculus)

I. Toxic Portion of Plant

A. Seed

II. Symptoms (some or all may be present)

A. Digestive upset

B. Depression or excitement

C. Dilated pupils

D. Paralysis

E. Coma with possible death

III. First Aid

A. If your cat is alert, induce vomiting.

B. Call your veterinarian immediately.

C. Observe for symptoms.

BUDDHIST PINE (Podocarpus)

I. Toxic Portion of Plant

A. All parts

II. Symptom

A. Severe digestive upset

III. First Aid

A. If your cat is alert, induce vomiting.

B. Call your veterinarian immediately.

C. Observe for symptoms.

BUTTERCUP (Ranunculus)

I. Toxic Portion of Plant

    A. Top growth

II. Symptom

    A. Digestive upset

III. First Aid

    A. If your cat is alert, induce vomiting.

    B. Call your veterinarian immediately.

    C. Observe for symptoms.

CALADIUM

I. Toxic Portion of Plant

    A. Leaves

    B. Stems

    C. Stalks

    D. Plant cells contain toxic calcium oxalate crystals.

II. Symptoms (some or all may be present)

    A. Digestive upset

    B. Irritation of mouth with possible swelling of the throat

    C. Possible asphyxiation

    D. Central nervous system signs - tremors, seizures, staggering, loss of coordination, etc.

    E. Possible death

III. First Aid

    A. If your cat is alert, induce vomiting.

    B. Call your veterinarian immediately.

    C. Observe for symptoms.

CALAMONDIN ORANGE (Citrus mitis)

I. Toxic Portion of Plant

    A. Leaves

    B. Stems

    C.   Stalks

    D.   Plant cells contain toxic calcium oxalate crystals.

II. **Symptoms (some or all may be present)**

    A.   Digestive upset

    B.   Irritation of mouth with possible swelling of the throat

    C.   Possible asphyxiation

    D.   Central nervous system signs - tremors, seizures, staggering, loss of coordination, etc.

    E.   Possible death

III. **First Aid**

    A.   If your cat is alert, induce vomiting.

    B.   Call your veterinarian immediately.

    C.   Observe for symptoms.

CALLA LILY (Zantedeschia)

I. **Toxic Portion of Plant**

    A.   Leaves

    B.   Stems

    C.   Stalks

    D.   Plant cells contain toxic calcium oxalate crystals.

II. **Symptoms (some or all may be present)**

    A.   Digestive upset

    B.   Irritation of mouth with possible swelling of the throat

    C.   Possible asphyxiation

    D.   Central nervous system signs - tremors, seizures, staggering, loss of coordination, etc.

    E.   Possible death

III. **First Aid**

    A.   If your cat is alert, induce vomiting.

    B.   Call your veterinarian immediately.

    C.   Observe for symptoms.

CASTOR BEAN (Ricinus communis)

I. **Toxic Portion of Plant**
  A. All parts
  B. Seeds are especially toxic.
  C. One leaf or seed may be deadly.

II. **Symptoms (some or all may be present)**
  A. Digestive upset
  B. Excess thirst
  C. Irritation of mouth and throat
  D. Liver and kidney damage
  E. Central nervous system signs - tremors, staggering, loss of coordination, etc.
  F. Seizures
  G. Possible death

III. **First Aid**
  A. If your cat is alert, induce vomiting.
  B. Call your veterinarian immediately.
  C. Observe for symptoms.

CERIMAN (Monstera deliciosa)

See Philodendron on page 220

CHARMING DIEFFENBACHIA (Dieffenbachia amoena)

See Dumb Cane on page 198

CHERRY (Prunus)

I. **Toxic Portion of Plant**
  A. Leaves and stems contain cyanide.
  B. Dried, withering leaves are most toxic.

II. **Symptoms (some or all may be present)**

A. Rapid breathing
B. Dilated pupils
C. Red gums
D. Shock
III. **First Aid**
   A. If your cat is alert, induce vomiting.
   B. Call your veterinarian immediately.
   C. Observe for symptoms.

CHRISTMAS ROSE (Helleborus niger)

I. **Toxic Portion of Plant**
   A. All parts
II. **Symptoms (some or all may be present)**
   A. Digestive upset
   B. Bloody diarrhea
   C. Seizures
   D. Disorientation
III. **First Aid**
   A. If your cat is alert, induce vomiting.
   B. Call your veterinarian immediately.
   C. Observe for symptoms.

CHRYSANTHEMUM

I. **Toxic Portion of Plant**
   A. All parts
II. **Symptom**
   A. Irritation of mucus membranes and any skin that comes in contact with the plant's resin.
III. **First Aid**
   A. Feed milk to your cat.
   B. Wash irritated skin with soap and water.
   C. Call your veterinarian immediately.
   D. Observe for symptoms.

CINERARIA (Senecio)

I. **Toxic Portion of Plant**
   A.   All parts
II. **Symptoms (some or all may be present)**
   A.   Digestive upset
   B.   Depression
   C.   Dark/muddy gum color
   D.   Liver damage
III. **First Aid**
   A.   If your cat is alert, induce vomiting.
   B.   Call your veterinarian immediately.
   C.   Observe for symptoms.

COLOCASIA

See Elephant's Ear on page 199

CORDATUM (Philodendron oxycardium)

I. **Toxic Portion of Plant**
   A.   Leaves
   B.   Stems
   C.   Stalks
   D.   Plant cells contain toxic calcium oxalate crystals.
II. **Symptoms (some or all may be present)**
   A.   Digestive upset
   B.   Irritation of mouth with possible swelling of the throat
   C.   Possible asphyxiation
   D.   Central nervous system signs - tremors, seizures, staggering, loss of coordination, etc.
   E.   Possible death
III. **First Aid**
   A.   If your cat is alert, induce vomiting.
   B.   Call your veterinarian immediately.

C.   Observe for symptoms.

CORN (CORNSTALK) PLANT (Dracaena fragrans massangeana)

I.   **Toxic Portion of Plant**

    A.   All parts

II.   **Symptoms (some or all may be present)**

    A.   Digestive upset

    B.   Dilated pupils

    C.   Difficult breathing

    D.   Drooling

    E.   Abdominal pain

III. **First Aid**

    A.   If your cat is alert, induce vomiting.

    B.   Call your veterinarian immediately.

    C.   Observe for symptoms.

CORYDALIS

I.   **Toxic Portion of Plant**

    A.   Top growth

    B.   Corms

II.   **Symptoms (some or all may be present)**

    A.   Digestive upset

    B.   Irritation of mouth with possible swelling of the throat

    C.   Possible asphyxiation

    D.   Central nervous system signs - tremors, seizures, staggering, loss of coordination, etc.

    E.   Possible death

III. **First Aid**

    A.   If your cat is alert, induce vomiting.

    B.   Call your veterinarian immediately.

    C.   Observe for symptoms.

CROTALARIA

I. **Toxic Portion of Plant**
   A. Seeds (plus other parts may also cause a toxic reaction)
II. **Symptoms (some or all may be present)**
   A. Liver damage
   B. Digestive upset
   C. Birth defects in offspring
III. **First Aid**
   A. If your cat is alert, induce vomiting.
   B. Call your veterinarian immediately.
   C. Observe for symptoms.

CROTON

I. **Toxic Portion of Plant**
   A. All parts
   B. Seeds are especially toxic.
   C. One leaf or seed may be deadly.
II. **Symptoms (some or all may be present)**
   A. Digestive upset
   B. Liver and kidney damage
   C. Central nervous system signs - tremors, seizures, staggering, loss of coordination, etc.
   D. Possible death
III. **First Aid**
   A. If your cat is alert, induce vomiting.
   B. Call your veterinarian immediately.
   C. Observe for symptoms.

CROWFOOT FAMILY

See Buttercup on page 188

CROWN OF THORNS (Euphorbia milii)

I. **Toxic Portion of Plant**
   A. All parts
II. **Symptoms (one or both may be present)**
   A. Digestive upset
   B. Skin irritation
III. **First Aid**
   A. If your cat is alert, induce vomiting.
   B. Call your veterinarian immediately.
   C. Observe for symptoms.

CUBAN LAUREL (Ficus)

I. **Toxic Portion of Plant**
   A. All parts
II. **Symptom**
   A. Digestive upset
III. **First Aid**
   A. If your cat is alert, induce vomiting.
   B. Call your veterinarian immediately.
   C. Observe for symptoms.

CYCAD (Cycas)

I. **Toxic Portion of Plant**
   A. All parts
II. **Symptoms (some or all may be present)**
   A. Digestive upset
   B. Black stools
   C. Internal bleeding
   D. Bruising
   E. Liver damage and jaundice - yellow hue to skin and gums
III. **First Aid**
   A. If your cat is alert, induce vomiting.

195

B. Call your veterinarian immediately.

C. Observe for symptoms.

CYCLAMEN

I. Toxic Portion of Plant

A. All parts

II. Symptoms (one or both may be present)

A. Digestive upset

B. Death

III. First Aid

A. If your cat is alert, induce vomiting.

B. Call your veterinarian immediately.

C. Observe for symptoms.

DAFFODIL (Narcissus)

I. Toxic Portion of Plant

A. Bulb is most toxic.

II. Symptoms (some or all may be present)

A. Digestive upset

B. Seizures

C. Shaking

D. Weakness

E. Irregular heart beats

F. Excitement followed by depression, then coma

G. Possible death

III. First Aid

A. If your cat is alert, induce vomiting.

B. Call your veterinarian immediately.

C. Observe for symptoms.

DAPHNE

I. **Toxic Portion of Plant**
    A. All parts
II. **Symptoms (some or all may be present)**
    A. Digestive upset
    B. Heart failure
    C. Excitement or depression
III. **First Aid**
    A. If your cat is alert, induce vomiting.
    B. Call your veterinarian immediately.
    C. Observe for symptoms.

DEATH CAMAS (Zigadenus)

I. **Toxic Portion of Plant**
    A. Bulb is most toxic.
II. **Symptoms (some or all may be present)**
    A. Digestive upset
    B. Excitement followed by depression, then coma
    C. Possible death
III. **First Aid**
    A. If your cat is alert, induce vomiting.
    B. Call your veterinarian immediately.
    C. Observe for symptoms.

DEVIL'S IVY

See Philodendron on page 220

DRACAENA PALM

See Corn Plant on page 193

DRAGON TREE (Dracaena draco)
See Corn Plant on page 193

DUMB CANE (DIEFFENBACHIA)

I. Toxic Portion of Plant
   A. Leaves
   B. Stems
   C. Stalks
   D. Plant cells contain toxic calcium oxalate crystals.

II. Symptoms (some or all may be present)
   A. Digestive upset
   B. Irritation of mouth with possible swelling of the throat
   C. Possible asphyxiation
   D. Central nervous system signs - tremors, seizures, staggering, loss of coordination, etc.
   E. Possible death

III. First Aid
   A. If your cat is alert, induce vomiting.
   B. Call your veterinarian immediately.
   C. Observe for symptoms.

EASTER LILY (Lilium longiflorum)

I. Toxic Portion of Plant
   A. All parts

II. Symptoms (some or all may be present)
   A. Kidney failure
   B. Digestive upset
   C. Weakness

III. First Aid
   A. If your cat is alert, induce vomiting.
   B. Call your veterinarian immediately.
   C. Observe for symptoms.

EGGPLANT

I. **Toxic Portion of Plant**
   A. Leaves
   B. Stems
   C. Stalks
   D. Sprouts
   E. Fruit is edible.

II. **Symptoms (some or all may be present)**
   A. Digestive upset
   B. Heart failure
   C. Depression/drowsiness
   D. Drooling
   E. Dilated pupils

III. **First Aid**
   A. If your cat is alert, induce vomiting.
   B. Call your veterinarian immediately.
   C. Observe for symptoms.

ELAINE CODIAEUM (Elaine)

See Croton on page 194

ELEPHANT'S EAR (Colocasia esculenta)

I. **Toxic Portion of Plant**
   A. Leaves
   B. Stems
   C. Stalks
   D. Plant cells contain toxic calcium oxalate crystals.

II. **Symptoms (some or all may be present)**
   A. Digestive upset
   B. Irritation of mouth with possible swelling of the throat
   C. Possible asphyxiation
   D. Central nervous system signs - tremors, seizures,

staggering, loss of coordination, etc.

    E.   Possible death

III. **First Aid**

    A.   If your cat is alert, induce vomiting.

    B.   Call your veterinarian immediately.

    C.   Observe for symptoms.

EMERALD FEATHER (Asparagus sprengeri)

See Asparagus Fern on page 231

ENGLISH IVY (Hedera helix)

I. **Toxic Portion of Plant**

    A.   All parts

    B.   Contains a saponic glycoside

II. **Symptoms (some or all may be present)**

    A.   Digestive upset

    B.   Excitability

    C.   Difficult breathing

    D.   Drooling

    E.   Fever

    F.   Increased thirst

    G.   Dilated pupils

    H.   Weakness

    I.   Staggering

III. **First Aid**

    A.   If your cat is alert, induce vomiting.

    B.   Call your veterinarian immediately.

    C.   Observe for symptoms.

EXOTICA PERFECTION DIEFFENBACHIA (Dieffenbachia exotica)

See Dumb Cane on page 198

FAVA BEAN (Vicia faba)

I. **Toxic Portion of Plant**

    A. Seeds (plus other parts may also cause a toxic reaction)

II. **Symptoms (some or all may be present)**

    A. Liver damage

    B. Digestive upset

    C. Birth defects in offspring

III. **First Aid**

    A. If your cat is alert, induce vomiting.

    B. Call your veterinarian immediately.

    C. Observe for symptoms.

FIDDLE-LEAF FIG (Ficus lyrata)

I. **Toxic Portion of Plant**

    A. All parts

II. **Symptoms (one or both may be present)**

    A. Skin irritation in some cats upon contact

    B. Digestive upset

III. **First Aid**

    A. If your cat is alert, induce vomiting.

    B. Call your veterinarian immediately.

    C. Observe for symptoms.

FINGER CHERRY (Rhodomyrtus macrocarpa)

I. **Toxic Portion of Plant**

A. Fruit
II. **Symptom**
   A. Blindness (may be complete and permanent)
III. **First Aid**
   A. If your cat is alert, induce vomiting.
   B. Call your veterinarian immediately.
   C. Observe for symptoms.

FLORIDA BEAUTY (Dracaena)

See Corn Plant on page 193

FOXGLOVE (Digitalis)

I. **Toxic Portion of Plant**
   A. All parts
   B. Seeds especially
II. **Symptoms (some or all may be present)**
   A. Digestive upset
   B. Central nervous system signs - tremors, seizures, staggering, loss of coordination, etc.
   C. Depression
   D. Collapse
   E. Heart failure
   F. Possible death
III. **First Aid**
   A. If your cat is alert, induce vomiting.
   B. Call your veterinarian immediately.
   C. Observe for symptoms.

FRUIT-SALAD PLANT (Monstera deliciosa)

See Philodendron on page 220

GERMAN IVY (Senecio mikanioides)
See Cineraria on page 192

GIANT DUMB CANE (Dieffenbachia amoena)
See Dumb Cane on page 198

GLACIER IVY (Hedera helix glacier)
See English Ivy on page 200

GOLD DIEFFENBACHIA (Dieffenbachia picta rudolph roehrs)
See Dumb Cane on page 198

GOLD DUST DRACAENA (Dracaena godseffiana)
See Corn Plant on page 193

GOLDEN POTHOS (Epipremnum aureum)
See Philodendron on page 220

GREEN GOLD NEPHTHYTIS (Syngonium podophyllum)
See Philodendron on page 220

GROUND CHERRY

I. **Toxic Portion of Plant**
   A. Leaves
   B. Stems
   C. Stalks
   D. Sprouts
   E. Fruit is edible.

II. **Symptoms (some or all may be present)**
   A. Digestive upset
   B. Drowsiness
   C. Weakness
   D. Drooling
   E. Shaking
   F. Paralysis
   G. Coma

III. **First Aid**
   A. If your cat is alert, induce vomiting.
   B. Call your veterinarian immediately.
   C. Observe for symptoms.

HEMLOCK (Conium maculatum)

I. **Toxic Portion of Plant**
   A. All parts

II. **Symptoms (some or all may be present)**
   A. Central nervous system signs - tremors, seizures, staggering, loss of coordination, etc.
   B. Depression

III. **First Aid**
   A. If your cat is alert, induce vomiting.
   B. Call your veterinarian immediately.
   C. Observe for symptoms.

HOLLY (Ilex)

I. **Toxic Portion of Plant**
    A. Berries
II. **Symptoms (one or both may be present)**
    A. Digestive upset
    B. Central nervous system depression
III. **First Aid**
    A. If your cat is alert, induce vomiting.
    B. Call your veterinarian immediately.
    C. Observe for symptoms.

HORSE BEAN (Vicia faba)
See Fava Bean on page 201

HORSEHEAD PHILODENDRON (Philodendron bipinnatifidum)
See Philodendron on page 220

HURRICANE PLANT (Monstera deliciosa)
See Philodendron on page 220

HYDRANGEA

I. **Toxic Portion of Plant**
    A. All parts
    B. Plants contain cyanide properties.
II. **Symptoms (some or all may be present)**
    A. Dizziness
    B. Increased breathing
    C. Seizures
III. **First Aid**

A. If your cat is alert, induce vomiting.

B. Call your veterinarian immediately.

C. Observe for symptoms.

INDIAN LAUREL (Ficus retusa nitida)

See Fiddle-leaf Fig on page 201

INDIAN TOBACCO (Lobelia inflata)

I. **Toxic Portion of Plant**

A. All parts

II. **Symptoms (some or all may be present)**

A. Digestive upset

B. Tremors

C. Stupor

D. Constricted pupils

E. Depression

III. **First Aid**

A. If your cat is alert, induce vomiting.

B. Call your veterinarian immediately.

C. Observe for symptoms.

INDIA RUBBER PLANT (Ficus elastica decora)

See Fiddle-leaf Fig on page 201

IRIS

I. **Toxic Portion of Plant**

A. Root

II. **Symptom**

A. Digestive upset

III. First Aid
   A. If your cat is alert, induce vomiting.
   B. Call your veterinarian immediately.
   C. Observe for symptoms.

JANET CRAIG DRACAENA (Dracaena deremensis Janet Craig)
See Corn Plant on page 193

JAPANESE YEW (Taxus cuspidata)

I. Toxic Portion of Plant
   A. All parts
   B. Berries

II. Symptoms (some or all may be present)
   A. Digestive upset
   B. Heart failure
   C. Shaking
   D. Difficult breathing
   E. Excitement or depression

III. First Aid
   A. If your cat is alert, induce vomiting.
   B. Call your veterinarian immediately.
   C. Observe for symptoms.

JAVA BEAN

I. Toxic Portion of Plant
   A. Seeds (plus other parts may also cause a toxic reaction)

II. Symptoms (some or all may be present)
   A. Liver damage
   B. Digestive upset
   C. Birth defects in offspring

207

III. First Aid
    A.   If your cat is alert, induce vomiting.
    B.   Call your veterinarian immediately.
    C.   Observe for symptoms.

JERUSALEM CHERRY (Solanum pseudocapsicum)

I. Toxic Portion of Plant
    A.   Berries (plus other parts may also cause a toxic reaction)

II. Symptoms (some or all may be present)
    A.   Digestive upset
    B.   Ulceration of the digestive tract
    C.   Seizures
    D.   Depression
    E.   Shaking
    F.   Drooling
    G.   Paralysis
    H.   Coma

III. First Aid
    A.   If your cat is alert, induce vomiting.
    B.   Call your veterinarian immediately.
    C.   Observe for symptoms.

JESSAMINE (Jasminum)

I. Toxic Portion of Plant
    A.   All parts

II. Symptoms (some or all may be present)
    A.   Weakness
    B.   Seizures
    C.   Difficult breathing and/or respiratory failure

III. First Aid
    A.   If your cat is alert, induce vomiting.

B. Call your veterinarian immediately.
C. Observe for symptoms.

JIMSONWEED (Datura stramonium)

I. **Toxic Portion of Plant**
   A. All parts
   B. Seeds are especially toxic.
II. **Symptoms (some or all may be present)**
   A. Digestive upset
   B. Disorientation
   C. Abnormal thirst
   D. Coma
   E. Possible death
III. **First Aid**
   A. If your cat is alert, induce vomiting.
   B. Call your veterinarian immediately.
   C. Observe for symptoms.

JONQUIL (Narcissus jonquilla)

I. **Toxic Portion of Plant**
   A. Bulb is most toxic.
II. **Symptoms (some or all may be present)**
   A. Digestive upset
   B. Excitement followed by depression, then coma
   C. Possible death
III. **First Aid**
   A. If your cat is alert, induce vomiting.
   B. Call your veterinarian immediately.
   C. Observe for symptoms.

KALANCHOE

I. **Toxic Portion of Plant**
    A.   All parts
II. **Symptom**
    A.   Digestive upset
III. **First Aid**
    A.   If your cat is alert, induce vomiting.
    B.   Call your veterinarian immediately.
    C.   Observe for symptoms.

LACY TREE PHILODENDRON (Philodendron selloum)

See Philodendron on page 220

LARKSPUR (Delphinium)

I. **Toxic Portion of Plant**
    A.   Flowers
    B.   Seeds
II. **Symptoms (some or all may be present)**
    A.   Digestive upset
    B.   Central nervous system signs - tremors, seizures, staggering, loss of coordination, etc.
    C.   Depression
    D.   Collapse
    E.   Heart failure
    F.   Possible death
III. **First Aid**
    A.   If your cat is alert, induce vomiting.
    B.   Call your veterinarian immediately.
    C.   Observe for symptoms.

LAUREL

I. **Toxic Portion of Plant**
    A. All parts

II. **Symptoms (some or all may be present)**
    A. Digestive upset
    B. Tearing
    C. Discharge from nose
    D. Drooling
    E. Seizures
    F. Slow heart rate
    G. Paralysis

III. **First Aid**
    A. If your cat is alert, induce vomiting.
    B. Call your veterinarian immediately.
    C. Observe for symptoms.

LILY OF THE VALLEY (Convallaria majalis)

I. **Toxic Portion of Plant**
    A. Bulb is most toxic.

II. **Symptoms (some or all may be present)**
    A. Digestive upset
    B. Excitement followed by depression, then coma
    C. Staggering
    D. Irregular heartbeat
    E. Possible death

III. **First Aid**
    A. If your cat is alert, induce vomiting.
    B. Call your veterinarian immediately.
    C. Observe for symptoms.

LOCO WEEDS

I. **Toxic Portion of Plant**
  A.   Seeds (plus other parts may also cause a toxic reaction)

II. **Symptoms (some or all may be present)**
  A.   Liver damage
  B.   Digestive upset
  C.   Central nervous system signs - tremors, seizures, staggering, loss of coordination, etc.
  D.   Birth defects in offspring

III. **First Aid**
  A.   If your cat is alert, induce vomiting.
  B.   Call your veterinarian immediately.
  C.   Observe for symptoms.

LUPINES

I. **Toxic Portion of Plant**
  A.   Berries (plus other parts may also cause a toxic reaction)

II. **Symptoms (some or all may be present)**
  A.   Liver damage
  B.   Digestive upset
  C.   Birth defects in offspring
  D.   Paralysis
  E.   Seizures
  F.   Depressed breathing

III. **First Aid**
  A.   If your cat is alert, induce vomiting.
  B.   Call your veterinarian immediately.
  C.   Observe for symptoms.

MADAGASCAR DRAGON TREE
(Dracaena marginata)

See Corn Plant on page 193

MANCHINEEL (Hippomane mancinella)

I. **Toxic Portion of Plant**
    A. Sap (found in all plant parts)
    B. Fruit
II. **Symptoms (one or both may be present)**
    A. Skin irritation from contact with the sap
    B. Severe digestive problems (from fruit especially)
III. **First Aid**
    A. Feed milk to your cat if your cat has ingested the plant.
    B. Wash any irritated skin with soap and water.
    C. Call your veterinarian immediately.
    D. Observe for symptoms.

MARBLE QUEEN (Scindapsus aureus Marble Queen)

I. **Toxic Portion of Plant**
    A. All parts
II. **Symptoms (some or all may be present)**
    A. Digestive upset
    B. Depression
    C. Respiratory depression
III. **First Aid**
    A. If your cat is alert, induce vomiting.
    B. Call your veterinarian immediately.
    C. Observe for symptoms.

MARIJUANA (Cannabis sativa)

I. **Toxic Portion of Plant**
    A. All parts
II. **Symptoms (some or all may be present)**
    A. Digestive upset
    B. Depression

C.   Respiratory depression

III.   **First Aid**
   A.   If your cat is alert, induce vomiting.
   B.   Call your veterinarian immediately.
   C.   Observe for symptoms.

MAY APPLE (Podophyllum peltatum)

I.   **Toxic Portion of Plant**
   A.   Roots

II.   **Symptoms (some or all may be present)**
   A.   Digestive upset
   B.   Depression
   C.   Exhaustion
   D.   Coma
   E.   Possible death

III.   **First Aid**
   A.   If your cat is alert, induce vomiting.
   B.   Call your veterinarian immediately.
   C.   Observe for symptoms.

MEDICINE PLANT (Aloe vera)

I.   **Toxic Portion of Plant**
   A.   All parts

II.   **Symptoms (one or both may be present)**
   A.   Diarrhea
   B.   Urine may turn red

III.   **First Aid**
   A.   If your cat is alert, induce vomiting.
   B.   Call your veterinarian immediately.
   C.   Observe for symptoms.

MISTLETOE (Phoradendron flavescens)

I. **Toxic Portion of Plant**
    A. All parts
    B. Seeds are especially toxic.
II. **Symptoms (some or all may be present)**
    A. Digestive upset
    B. Depression
    C. Heart failure
    D. Exhaustion
    E. Coma
    F. Possible death
III. **First Aid**
    A. If your cat is alert, induce vomiting.
    B. Call your veterinarian immediately.
    C. Observe for symptoms.

MONKSHOOD (Aconitum)

I. **Toxic Portion of Plant**
    A. Flowers
    B. Seeds
II. **Symptoms (some or all may be present)**
    A. Digestive upset
    B. Central nervous system signs - tremors, seizures, staggering, loss of coordination, etc.
    C. Depression
    D. Collapse
    E. Heart failure
    F. Possible death
III. **First Aid**
    A. If your cat is alert, induce vomiting.
    B. Call your veterinarian immediately.
    C. Observe for symptoms.

MORNING GLORY (Ipomoea)

I. **Toxic Portion of Plant**
    A.   All parts
    B.   Seeds contain LSD-like compounds.

II. **Symptoms (one or both may be present)**
    A.   Digestive upset
    B.   Hallucinations

III. **First Aid**
    A.   If your cat is alert, induce vomiting.
    B.   Call your veterinarian immediately.
    C.   Observe for symptoms.

MOTHER-IN-LAW PLANT (Dieffenbachia)

See Dumb Cane on page 198

MUSHROOMS

I. **Toxicity**
    A.   Many species of mushrooms and toadstools are poisonous, especially the Amanita species.

II. **Symptoms (some or all may be present)**
    A.   Digestive upset
    B.   Drooling
    C.   Constricted or dilated pupils
    D.   Shaking/shivering/muscle spasms
    E.   Weakness
    F.   Irregular heartbeat
    G.   Liver damage
    H.   Possible blood in urine
    I.   Possible coma and death

III. **First Aid**
    A.   Identify the mushroom the cat has ingested. If the

mushroom cannot be identified, obtain a sample of the fungus. Plants can be identified by veterinarians and by plant identification books.

    B.   If you suspect that the mushroom is poisonous and your cat is alert, induce vomiting and call a veterinarian.

    C.   Observe for symptoms.

NARCISSUS

I.   **Toxic Portion of Plant**

    A.   Bulb is most toxic.

II.   **Symptoms (some or all may be present)**

    A.   Digestive upset

    B.   Excitement followed by depression, then coma

    C.   Seizures

    D.   Shaking/shivering

    E.   Weakness

    F.   Irregular heartbeat

    G.   Possible death

III.   **First Aid**

    A.   If your cat is alert, induce vomiting.

    B.   Call your veterinarian immediately.

    C.   Observe for symptoms.

NEEDLEPOINT IVY (Hedera helix needlepoint)

See English Ivy on page 200

NIGHTSHADE (Solanum)

I.   **Toxic Portion of Plant**

    A.   All parts

    B.   Berries are also toxic.

II. Symptoms (some or all may be present)
A. Digestive upset
B. Heart failure
C. Depression/drowsiness
D. Drooling
E. Dilated pupils
III. First Aid
A. If your cat is alert, induce vomiting.
B. Call your veterinarian immediately.
C. Observe for symptoms.

OLEANDER (Nerium oleander)

I. Toxic Portion of Plant
A. All parts
II. Symptoms (some or all may be present)
A. Digestive upset
B. Heart failure
C. Excitement or depression
D. Oral irritation
E. Decreased body temperature
III. First Aid
A. If your cat is alert, induce vomiting.
B. Call your veterinarian immediately.
C. Observe for symptoms.

ONION (Allium)

I. Toxic Portion of Plant
A. All parts
II. Symptoms (one or both may be present)
A. Digestive upset
B. Weakness from hemolytic anemia
III. First Aid

A. If your cat is alert, induce vomiting.

B. Call your veterinarian immediately.

C. Observe for symptoms.

PANDA (Philodendron panduraeformae)
See Philodendron on page 220

PEA (Lathyrus)
I. Toxic Portion of Plant
   A. All parts
   B. Seeds especially
II. Symptoms (some or all may be present)
   A. Seizures
   B. Paralysis
   C. Depressed breathing
III. First Aid
   A. If your cat is alert, induce vomiting.
   B. Call your veterinarian immediately.
   C. Observe for symptoms.

PEACE LILY (Spathiphyllum)
See Philodendron on page 220

PENCIL CACTUS (Euphorbia tirucalli)
I. Toxic Portion of Plant
   A. All parts
II. Symptoms (one or both may be present)
   A. Digestive upset
   B. Irritation of skin/blistering
III. First Aid

A. If your cat is alert, induce vomiting.
B. Call your veterinarian immediately.
C. Observe for symptoms.

PEONY (Paeonia)

I. **Toxic Portion of Plant**
   A. Flowers
   B. Seeds
II. **Symptoms (some or all may be present)**
   A. Digestive upset
   B. Central nervous system signs - tremors, seizures, staggering, loss of coordination, etc.
   C. Depression
   D. Collapse
   E. Heart failure
   F. Possible death
III. **First Aid**
   A. If your cat is alert, induce vomiting.
   B. Call your veterinarian immediately.
   C. Observe for symptoms.

PHILODENDRON

I. **Toxic Portion of Plant**
   A. All parts
II. **Symptoms (some or all may be present)**
   A. Digestive upset
   B. Irritation of mouth with possible swelling of the throat
   C. Possible asphyxiation
   D. Central nervous system signs - tremors, seizures, staggering, loss of coordination, etc.
   E. Possible death
III. **First Aid**

A. If your cat is alert, induce vomiting.
B. Call your veterinarian immediately.
C. Observe for symptoms.

PLUMOSA FERN
See Asparagus Fern on page 231

POINSETTIA (Euphorbia pulcherrima)

I. Toxic Portion of Plant
   A. All parts
II. Symptoms (one or both may be present)
   A. Digestive upset
   B. Irritation to the mouth and stomach
III. First Aid
   A. If your cat is alert, induce vomiting.
   B. Call your veterinarian immediately.
   C. Observe for symptoms.

POKEWEED (Phytolacca)

I. Toxic Portion of Plant
   A. Roots
II. Symptoms (some or all may be present)
   A. Digestive upset
   B. Depression
   C. Exhaustion
   D. Coma
   E. Possible death
III. First Aid
   A. If your cat is alert, induce vomiting.
   B. Call your veterinarian immediately.
   C. Observe for symptoms.

POTATO

I. **Toxic Portion of Plant**

    A. Leaves

    B. Stems

    C. Stalks

    D. Sprouts

    E. Tuber is edible.

II. **Symptoms (some or all may be present)**

    A. Digestive upset

    B. Heart failure

    C. Depression/drowsiness

    D. Drooling

    E. Dilated pupils

III. **First Aid**

    A. If your cat is alert, induce vomiting.

    B. Call your veterinarian immediately.

    C. Observe for symptoms.

POTHOS (Scindapsus)

See Philodendron on page 220

PRECATORY BEAN (Abrus precatorius)

I. **Toxic Portion of Plant**

    A. Beans are very poisonous.

II. **Symptoms (some or all may be present)**

    A. Digestive upset

    B. Fever

    C. Staggering

    D. Death

III. **First Aid**

    A. If your cat is alert, induce vomiting.

    B. Call your veterinarian immediately.

C.   Observe for symptoms.

PRIMROSE (Primula)

I.   **Toxic Portion of Plant**
    A.   All parts

II.   **Symptom**
    A.   Digestive upset

III. **First Aid**
    A.   If your cat is alert, induce vomiting.
    B.   Call your veterinarian immediately.
    C.   Observe for symptoms.

PRIVET

I.   **Toxic Portion of Plant**
    A.   Berries
    B.   Leaves

II.   **Symptoms (one or both may be present)**
    A.   Digestive upset
    B.   Kidney damage

III. **First Aid**
    A.   If your cat is alert, induce vomiting.
    B.   Call your veterinarian immediately.
    C.   Observe for symptoms.

RAYLESS GOLDENROD

I.   **Toxic Portion of Plant**
    A.   All parts

II.   **Symptoms (some or all may be present)**
    A.   Digestive upset
    B.   Weakness
    C.   Constipation

D.   Seizures
E.   Liver damage/failure
F.   Kidney damage

III.   First Aid

A.   If your cat is alert, induce vomiting.
B.   Call your veterinarian immediately.
C.   Observe for symptoms.

RED EMERALD (Philodendron Red Emerald)

See Philodendron on page 220

RED-MARGINED DRACAENA (Dracaena marginata)

See Corn Plant on page 193

RED PRINCESS (Philodendron Red Princess)

See Philodendron on page 220

RHODODENDRON

See Azalea on page 185

RIBBON PLANT (Dracaena sanderiana)

See Corn Plant on page 193

SAGO PALM (Cycas)

See Cycad on page 195

SCHEFFLERA (Brassaia actinophylla)

See Philodendron on page 220

SNOW-ON-THE-MOUNTAIN (Euphorbia marginata)

I. **Toxic Portion of Plant**
   A. All parts
   B. Seeds are especially toxic.
   C. One leaf or seed may be deadly.
II. **Symptoms (some or all may be present)**
   A. Digestive upset
   B. Liver and kidney damage
   C. Central nervous system signs - tremors, seizures, staggering, loss of coordination, etc.
   D. Possible death
III. **First Aid**
   A. If your cat is alert, induce vomiting.
   B. Call your veterinarian immediately.
   C. Observe for symptoms.

STAR-OF-BETHLEHEM

I. **Toxic Portion of Plant**
   A. Bulb is most toxic.
II. **Symptoms (some or all may be present)**
   A. Digestive upset
   B. Excitement followed by depression, then coma
   C. Possible death
III. **First Aid**
   A. If your cat is alert, induce vomiting.
   B. Call your veterinarian immediately.
   C. Observe for symptoms.

STRING OF PEARLS/BEADS (Senecio rowleyanus)

I.   **Toxic Portion of Plant**
   A.   All parts
II. **Symptoms (one or both may be present)**
   A.   Digestive upset
   B.   Irregular heartbeat
III. **First Aid**
   A.   If your cat is alert, induce vomiting.
   B.   Call your veterinarian immediately.
   C.   Observe for symptoms.

STRIPED DRACAENA (Dracaena deremensis Warnickei)

See Corn Plant on page 193

SWEETHEART IVY (Hedera helix sweetheart)

See English Ivy on page 200

TARO

See Elephant's Ear on page 199

TARO VINE (Scindapsus aureus)

See Philodendron on page 220

TAXUS (Yew)

I.   **Toxic Portion of Plant**

A. All parts

B. Especially berries

II. Symptoms (some or all may be present)

A. Digestive upset

B. Excitement or depression

C. Heart failure

III. First Aid

A. If your cat is alert, induce vomiting.

B. Call your veterinarian immediately.

C. Observe for symptoms.

TOADSTOOLS

I. Toxicity

A. Many species of toadstools and mushrooms are poisonous, especially the Amanita species.

II. Symptoms (some or all may be present)

A. Digestive upset

B. Drooling

C. Constricted or dilated pupils

D. Shaking/shivering/muscle spasms

E. Weakness

F. Irregular heartbeat

G. Liver damage

H. Possible blood in urine

I. Possible coma and death

III. First Aid

A. If your cat is alert, induce vomiting and call a veterinarian.

B. Identify the toadstool the cat has ingested. If the toadstool cannot be identified, obtain a sample of the fungus. Plants can be identified by veterinarians and by plant identification books.

C. Observe for symptoms.

TOMATO (Lycopersicon)

I. **Toxic Portion of Plant**
- A. Leaves
- B. Stems
- C. Stalks
- D. Fruit is edible.

II. **Symptoms (some or all may be present)**
- A. Digestive upset
- B. Depression/drowsiness
- C. Drooling
- D. Dilated pupils
- E. Heart failure

III. **First Aid**
- A. If your cat is alert, induce vomiting.
- B. Call your veterinarian immediately.
- C. Observe for symptoms.

VARIABLE DIEFFENBACHIA (Dieffenbachia picta)

See Dumb Cane on page 198

VARIEGATED RUBBER PLANT (Ficus elastica variegata)

See Fiddle-leaf Fig on page 199

WATER HEMLOCK (Cicuta)

I. **Toxic Portion of Plant**
- A. Tuber mostly

II. **Symptoms (one or both may be present)**
- A. Central nervous system signs - tremors, seizures,

staggering, loss of coordination, etc.

    B.   Seizures

III. First Aid

    A.   If your cat is alert, induce vomiting.

    B.   Call your veterinarian immediately.

    C.   Observe for symptoms.

WEEPING FIG (Ficus benjamina)

See Fiddle-leaf Fig on page 199

WILD ACONITE

I.   Toxic Portion of Plant

    A.   All parts

II.   Symptoms (some or all may be present)

    A.   Digestive upset with bloody diarrhea

    B.   Disorientation

    C.   Staggering

    D.   Difficulty breathing

    E.   Seizures

    F.   Coma and possible death

III. First Aid

    A.   If your cat is alert, induce vomiting.

    B.   Call your veterinarian immediately.

    C.   Observe for symptoms.

WISTERIA

I.   Toxic Portion of Plant

    A.   All parts

II.   Symptom

    A.   Digestive upset

III. First Aid

A.   If your cat is alert, induce vomiting.
B.   Call your veterinarian immediately.
C.   Observe for symptoms.

YEW (Taxus)

See Japanese Yew on page 207 or Taxus on page 226

PLANTS THAT CAUSE SKIN IRRITATION

I. List of Plants

A. Asparagus fern
B. Chrysanthemum resin
C. Manchineel sap
D. Poinsettia sap
E. Primrose leaves

II. First Aid

A. Wash affected area with soap and water.
B. Cleanse area with alcohol.

NONPOISONOUS PLANTS

I. A Warning

A. Even though many plants are not toxic, when ingested in quantity they can cause digestive upset. Also, even plants that are generally not considered to be poisonous can cause an allergic reaction that may be serious. Each cat is unique, and a plant that may cause no difficulties for one cat may be toxic for another.

II. Special Considerations

A. Plants may be sprayed with chemicals which can be toxic to cats.
B. Often a cat will eat plants when the cat feels ill from something else.

PART 6

—

OTHER POISONS

ACETAMINOPHEN (TYLENOL®) TOXICITY

Like many human drugs, Tylenol® is toxic to cats. In fact one capsule may be lethal if the cat does not receive veterinary treatment. No medications of any kind should be given to a cat without instructions from a veterinarian. And because cats are curious by nature, all drugs should be kept out of your cat's reach to prevent accidental ingestion.

I. Symptoms

A. Listlessness
B. Difficulty breathing
C. Vomiting and/or diarrhea
D. Dark-colored urine

II. First-Aid Materials

A. Hydrogen peroxide
B. Eyedropper

III. First Aid

A. If the pet is conscious, induce vomiting immediately by feeding the cat 1 teaspoon of hydrogen peroxide (mixed with 1 teaspoon milk if available). If the cat will not drink the mixture or if there is no milk available, then force-feed the cat the hydrogen peroxide using an eyedropper. If vomiting does not occur within 10 minutes, repeat the procedure twice.

B.   Contact a veterinarian for further treatment regardless of whether you are successful at inducing vomiting.

ACIDS AND ALKALIS

Acids and alkalis can be found in a wide variety of products. Acids include: sulfuric (found in auto batteries and metal cleaners and polishes), hydrochloric (in metal cleaners and polishes), nitric (in permanent wave neutralizer), oxalic (in cleaning solutions, bleach, and furniture and floor polishes and waxes), carbolic acid or phenol (in antiseptics and disinfectants). Alkalis include: sodium hydroxide/lye (in aquarium products, drain cleaners and small batteries), potassium hydroxide (in cuticle remover and some small batteries), sodium phosphate (in abrasive cleaners), sodium carbonate (in dye removers and dishwasher soap). In addition, there are milder alkalis found in ammonia and bleaches. Ingestion of acids or alkalis can cause severe internal irritation as well as external burns. Because these poisons are extreme irritants, **do not induce vomiting**.

I. Symptoms

A. Salivating
B. Vomiting
C. Diarrhea
D. Weakness

II. First-Aid Materials

A. Milk of Magnesia®
B. Lemon juice
C. Vinegar
D. Baking soda
E. Eyedropper

III. First Aid

A. **Do not induce vomiting.**
B. **For acid ingestion,** feed your cat 1 teaspoon Milk of Magnesia® using an eyedropper.
C. **For acid burns,** flush areas with copious amounts of water. Apply a paste of 1 part baking soda to 2 parts water to burns.
D. **For alkali ingestion,**
   (1) Mix 1/4 teaspoon vinegar with 1 teaspoon water and feed the mixture to your cat using an eyedropper, **or**
   (2) Feed your cat 1 teaspoon lemon juice using an eyedropper.
E. **For alkali burns,** flush the areas with copious amounts of water. Apply a solution of 1 cup vinegar to 4 cups water over areas.
F. Contact a veterinarian for additional instructions.

ANTIFREEZE TOXICITY

Antifreeze is a common poison to pets for three reasons: it is a commonly-used product, it is often improperly discarded, and it is sweet to the taste.

Antifreeze contains ethylene glycol which, when metabolized, causes kidney damage that is usually fatal. Even a small amount will cause severe illness or death. Because the toxin is rapidly absorbed, symptoms may appear as early as one hour after ingestion. Symptoms are vague and mimic those of many other conditions and diseases.

I.   Symptoms (some or all may be present)

A.   Increased thirst

B.   Vomiting and diarrhea

C.   Depression

D.   Loss of coordination

E.   The pet may show slight improvement in its condition before its kidneys fail.

II.   First-Aid Materials

A.   Hydrogen peroxide

B.   Liquor (e.g., vodka, whiskey, gin, rum)

C.   Eyedropper

III. First Aid

A. If an exposure is suspected, induce vomiting by feeding the cat
1 teaspoon of hydrogen peroxide (mixed with 1 teaspoon milk if
available). If the cat will not drink the mixture or if there is no
milk available, then force-feed the cat the hydrogen peroxide
using an eyedropper. If vomiting does not occur within
10 minutes, repeat the procedure up to two times.

B. Get immediate veterinary help.

C. If a veterinarian cannot be found, then when vomiting ceases or
if vomiting cannot be induced, use an eyedropper to feed the cat
1 tablespoon of liquor (e.g., vodka, whiskey, gin, rum) mixed
with 1 tablespoon of half and half cream. (If half and half
cream is not available, then use milk or water.) Wait 10 minutes,
and if there are no signs of depression or intoxication, administer
another 1/2 tablespoon of liquor mixed with 1/2 tablespoon of
half and half cream. (The ethanol in liquor competes with the
ethylene glycol metabolism decreasing the amounts that may
cause damage to the kidneys. It also promotes increased
urination to allow faster excretion of the poison.)

D. Seek veterinary attention for further treatment.

ARSENIC POISONING

Arsenic poisoning can occur in cats that ingest water or plants that have been contaminated with herbicides or pesticides containing arsenic. If your cat does ingest arsenic, early treatment is essential because arsenic is extremely toxic.

I. Symptoms (some or all may be present)

A. Abdominal pain
B. Weakness
C. Salivating
D. Vomiting
E. Diarrhea
F. Shaking
G. Staggering
H. Collapse
I. Death

II. First-Aid Materials

A. Hydrogen peroxide
B. Eyedropper
C. Raw egg whites

III. First Aid

A. If an exposure is suspected, induce vomiting by feeding the cat 1 teaspoon of hydrogen peroxide (mixed with 1 teaspoon milk if available). If the cat will not drink the mixture or if there is no milk available, then force-feed the cat the hydrogen peroxide using an eyedropper. If vomiting does not occur within 10 minutes, repeat the procedure up to two times.

B. Get immediate veterinary help.

C. If a veterinarian cannot be found, then when vomiting ceases or if vomiting cannot be induced, using an eyedropper slowly feed the cat 1 teaspoon of raw egg whites.

ASPIRIN TOXICITY

Many human drugs are toxic to cats, including aspirin. No medications should be given to a cat without specific instructions from a veterinarian. Also, cats are curious, and any drugs should be kept out of their reach to prevent accidental ingestion.

I. Symptoms (some or all may be present)

A. Depression
B. Digestive upset
C. Fever
D. Rapid breathing
E. Seizures
F. Shock
G. Long-term low-dose exposure may cause anemia, bleeding and liver damage.

II. First-Aid Materials

A. Hydrogen peroxide
B. Eyedropper

III. First Aid

A. If the pet is conscious, induce vomiting immediately by feeding the cat 1 teaspoon of hydrogen peroxide (mixed with 1 teaspoon milk if available). If the cat will not drink the mixture or if there is no milk available, then force-feed the cat the hydrogen peroxide using an eyedropper. If vomiting does not occur within 10 minutes, repeat the procedure twice.

B. Contact your veterinarian for further treatment, regardless of whether you have been successful at inducing vomiting.

CHOCOLATE TOXICITY

Chocolate contains a substance called theobromine which cannot be readily metabolized by cats. Even in small quantities, chocolate may be toxic to your cat.

I. Symptoms (some or all may be present)

A. Moderate to severe vomiting and diarrhea
B. Excitability and nervousness
C. Muscle tremors and/or seizures
D. Heart failure

II. First-Aid Materials

A. Hydrogen peroxide
B. Eyedropper

III. First Aid

A. If the ingestion has occurred within the previous 6 hours, immediately induce vomiting by feeding the cat 1 teaspoon of hydrogen peroxide (mixed with 1 teaspoon milk if available). If the cat will not drink the mixture or if there is no milk available, then force-feed the cat the hydrogen peroxide using an eyedropper. If vomiting does not occur within 10 minutes, repeat the procedure twice.
B. See a veterinarian for further monitoring and supportive care.

ETHYLENE GLYCOL TOXICITY

Ethylene glycol is a chemical found in automobile antifreeze. Unfortunately, cats find that antifreeze has a pleasant odor, and outdoor cats are therefore highly susceptible to ethylene glycol poisoning. When ethylene glycol is metabolized, it causes kidney damage that is usually fatal. Even a small amount will cause severe illness or death. Because the toxin is rapidly absorbed, symptoms may appear as early as one hour after ingestion. Symptoms are vague and mimic those of many other conditions and diseases.

I.   Symptoms (some or all may be present)

A.   Increased thirst
B.   Vomiting and diarrhea
C.   Depression
D.   Loss of coordination
E.   The cat may show slight improvement in its condition before its kidneys fail.

II.   First-Aid Materials

A.   Hydrogen peroxide
B.   Liquor (e.g., vodka, whiskey, gin, rum)
C.   Eyedropper

III. First Aid

A. If an exposure is suspected, induce vomiting by feeding the cat
    1 teaspoon of hydrogen peroxide (mixed with 1 teaspoon milk if
    available). If the cat will not drink the mixture or if there is no
    milk available, then force-feed the cat the hydrogen peroxide
    using an eyedropper. If vomiting does not occur within
    10 minutes, repeat the procedure up to two times.
B. Get immediate veterinary help.
C. If a veterinarian cannot be found, then when vomiting ceases or
    if vomiting cannot be induced, use an eyedropper to feed the cat
    1 tablespoon of liquor (e.g., vodka, whiskey, gin, rum) mixed
    with 1 tablespoon of half and half cream. (If half and half
    cream is not available, then use milk or water.) Wait 10 minutes,
    and if there are no signs of depression or intoxication, administer
    another 1/2 tablespoon of liquor mixed with 1/2 tablespoon of
    half and half cream. (The ethanol in liquor competes with the
    ethylene glycol metabolism decreasing the amounts that may
    cause damage to the kidneys. It also promotes increased
    urination to allow faster excretion of the poison.)
D. Seek veterinary attention for further treatment.

FLEA PRODUCT TOXICITY

Flea products are chemicals, and sometimes cats have reactions to them. It is important to follow the flea-product directions to minimize the risk to your cat. The relatively small risk associated with using flea products is justified, however, because fleas can spread parasites and infections, and they can cause fatal anemia.

I. Symptoms

A. Drooling longer than 20 minutes
B. Loss of appetite
C. Digestive upset
D. Seizures or muscle tremors (in severe cases)
E. Disorientation

II. First-Aid Materials

A. Shampoo that does not contain flea chemicals

III. First Aid

A. If chemicals have been applied to the cat, immediately wash off the product using shampoo and water. Repeat once.
B. See a veterinarian for an antidote, further monitoring, and supportive care.

IBUPROFEN TOXICITY

Ibuprofen is an anti-inflammatory drug that, for cats, is even more toxic than aspirin. Because ibuprofen is a common household medication, cats often have easy access to the drug. Never give any medications to a cat without the advice of a veterinarian.

I. Symptoms (some or all may be present)

A. Digestive upset
B. Bloody stool
C. Depression
D. Staggering
E. Increased thirst
F. Increased frequency of urination
G. Liver disease
H. Kidney disease
I. Seizures

II. First-Aid Materials

A. Hydrogen peroxide
B. Eyedropper

III. First Aid

A. If the pet is conscious, induce vomiting immediately by feeding the cat 1 teaspoon of hydrogen peroxide (mixed with 1 teaspoon milk if available). If the cat will not drink the mixture or if there is no milk available, then force-feed the cat the hydrogen peroxide using an eyedropper. If vomiting does not occur within 10 minutes, repeat the procedure twice.

B. Contact your veterinarian for further treatment regardless of whether you have been successful at inducing vomiting.

LEAD TOXICITY

Lead poisoning is becoming less common because of an increased awareness of its health hazards. Lead poisoning is seen more commonly in dogs than in cats because dogs tend to chew extraneous objects to a greater extent than do cats. Products like paint, plaster, caulking, linoleum, solder, improperly glazed dishes, fishing sinkers and golf balls sometimes contain lead.

I. Symptoms

A. Digestive upset
B. Loss of appetite
C. Personality/behavior change
D. Seizures and blindness (in severe cases)

II. First-Aid Materials

A. Hydrogen peroxide
B. Eyedropper
C. Raw egg white

III. First Aid

A. If the ingestion has occurred within the last 6 hours, immediately induce vomiting by feeding the cat 1 teaspoon of hydrogen peroxide (mixed with 1 teaspoon milk if available). If the cat will not drink the mixture or if there is no milk available, then force-feed the cat the hydrogen peroxide using an eyedropper.

If vomiting does not occur within 10 minutes, repeat the procedure twice.

B. After vomiting has stopped, or if you are unsuccessful at inducing vomiting, mix 1 raw egg white with 1 teaspoon of water. Feed the cat 1 teaspoon of this mixture slowly with an eyedropper.

C. See a veterinarian for further monitoring and supportive care.

PETROLEUM DISTILLATES

Petroleum distillates include gasoline, kerosene, paint thinner, lighter fluid, mineral spirits, diesel fuel, some household all-purpose lubricating oils (e.g., WD-40® and 3-IN-ONE® household oil) and petroleum-based insecticides (e.g., Raid®). Some furniture polishes and cleaners also contain petroleum distillates. If ingestion of petroleum distillates does occur, **do not induce vomiting.** Vomiting may cause the petroleum to become aspirated (i.e., breathed into the lungs), which will cause respiratory irritations and possibly pneumonia.

I. Symptoms (some or all may be present)

A. Salivation
B. Odor of petroleum
C. Difficulty breathing

II. First-Aid Materials

A. Any vegetable oil
B. Eyedropper

III. First Aid

A. Feed the cat 1 teaspoon of vegetable oil using an eyedropper.
B. Contact a veterinarian immediately.

RAT POISON

Rat poisons are laced in a grain base which intrigues cats. When a cat eats rat poison, the poison interferes with the cat's ability to make vitamin K. Vitamin K is essential in causing blood to clot, and without the vitamin, a cat will hemorrhage internally. Because the symptoms from rat poison take several days to appear, early treatment is essential if an exposure is even suspected.

I. Symptoms (some or all may be present)

A. None for several days
B. Weakness – frequently the first symptom
C. Pale, white or bruised gums
D. Bruises on the cat's body
E. Bloody urine and/or stools
F. Blue-green feces or vomitus – some rat baits contain a blue-green dye
G. Death – may occur within 24 hours from the time symptoms develop

II. First-Aid Materials

A. Hydrogen peroxide
B. Eyedropper

III. First Aid

A. If exposure has occurred within 6 hours, immediately induce vomiting by feeding the cat 1 teaspoon of hydrogen peroxide (mixed with 1 teaspoon milk if available). If the cat will not drink the mixture or if there is no milk available, then force-feed the cat the hydrogen peroxide using an eyedropper. If vomiting does not occur within 10 minutes, repeat the procedure twice.

B. Regardless of whether you have been able to induce vomiting, seek veterinary care immediately. Your veterinarian will prescribe vitamin K as an antidote and may also prescribe medicines to slow absorption of the poison.

SNAIL BAIT

Snail bait is poisonous to pets because it contains the chemical metaldehyde. This product, like rat poison, is made with a tasty base that attracts not only snails but also cats.

I.   Symptoms

A.   Loss of coordination
B.   Muscle tremors or convulsions
C.   Increased heart rate

II.   First-Aid Materials

A.   Hydrogen peroxide
B.   Eyedropper

III.   First Aid

A.   Induce vomiting if exposure is suspected. (Do not attempt to induce vomiting if the pet exhibits any loss of coordination or is having a seizure because the pet could aspirate vomit into its lungs.) Induce vomiting by feeding the cat 1 teaspoon of hydrogen peroxide (mixed with 1 teaspoon milk if available). If the cat will not drink the mixture or if there is no milk available, then force-feed the cat the hydrogen peroxide using an eyedropper. If vomiting does not occur within 10 minutes, repeat the procedure twice.
B.   Contact a veterinarian immediately.

STRYCHNINE POISONING

Strychnine is sometimes an ingredient in products sold to kill insects and rodents. The products are laced with a sweetener to attract the animal and generally contain enough strychnine that even ingestion of a small amount of the product will kill the pest. Unfortunately, strychnine is highly poisonous, and even a small amount will likely kill your cat. If your cat does ingest strychnine, immediate action is necessary.

I.   Symptoms

A.   Symptoms may appear within 2 hours of ingestion.
B.   The cat may appear to be apprehensive or nervous.
C.   Stiffness may develop, leading to severe seizures. These seizures can be provoked or exacerbated by external stimuli (e.g., noise, trauma, etc.).
D.   Exhaustion and death may shortly follow the onset of symptoms.

II.   First-Aid Materials

A.   Hydrogen peroxide
B.   Eyedropper

III. First Aid

A.   If the pet is conscious and alert, immediately induce vomiting by feeding the cat 1 teaspoon of hydrogen peroxide (mixed with 1 teaspoon milk if available). If the cat will not drink the mixture or if there is no milk available, then force-feed the cat the hydrogen peroxide using an eyedropper. If vomiting does not occur within 10 minutes, repeat the procedure twice.

B. To keep your cat from injuring itself during a seizure, block off access to stairways and move any objects or furniture that may cause injury. If a seizure does occur, see page 107 for additional instructions.

C. Keep the cat in a quiet environment.

D. Seek veterinary help.

YARD CHEMICALS

A variety of chemicals in fertilizers and pesticides can cause illness either from inhalation, contact or ingestion. Symptoms of illness may be delayed for days, but may be quite severe. Avoid exposing your cat to these toxins by keeping your cat indoors during and immediately after yard fertilization and spraying, and if you are using an insecticide indoors, keep your cat out of the room until the chemicals have dissipated. Never spray your cat with an insecticide that is not labeled specifically for use on cats.

I. Symptoms (some or all may be present)

A. Listlessness
B. Loss of appetite
C. Difficulty breathing
D. Vomiting
E. Diarrhea
F. Skin irritation from contact (typically the pads of the feet)

II. First Aid Materials

A. Shampoo

III. First Aid

A. If the cat gets chemicals on its fur, bathe the cat with cat shampoo (or any mild moisturizing shampoo if cat shampoo is not available). While restraining the cat, apply the shampoo and let it stand for 10 minutes before rinsing well.
B. Seek veterinary assistance for additional advice and treatment.

PART 7

—

DISEASES THAT CAN
BECOME EMERGENCIES

GENERAL INFORMATION

There are many diseases and conditions that are not emergencies but can develop into emergencies if untreated. All of the diseases and conditions discussed in Part 7 of this book call for veterinarian care to prevent a crisis from developing. Early treatment may result in complete cure, whereas lack of proper care can eventually lead to a crisis and possibly death.

Because your cat is unable to communicate effectively when there is a problem developing, always try to be aware of any changes in your cat's behavior, appearance or physical condition. If your cat has any history of any diseases or conditions that may become an emergency, ask your veterinarian for signs to look for that may indicate a return or worsening of the situation. If in doubt, always seek veterinary advice early rather than waiting until a more serious situation develops.

For additional information on prevention of emergencies see the chapter starting on page 8 and the Appendix on page 301.

DENTAL DISEASE

Dental-related emergencies can be avoided by providing your cat with regular veterinary dental care. A cat's teeth should be checked by a veterinarian for dental disease at least every six months. Dental disease can cause pain, discomfort, and infection in the cat's mouth, and if left untreated, it can be life-threatening. Any infection in the mouth can spread into the bloodstream where it can cause a variety of problems, including damage to the heart, liver and kidneys.

I. Symptoms of dental disease (some or all may be present)

A. Bad breath
B. Difficulty chewing
C. Brownish-yellow-green plaque buildup on teeth
D. Recessed, reddened gums
E. Sneezing
F. Swelling below eyes
G. Drooling

II. Home care

A. Check the cat's teeth at home once weekly by pulling back the corner of the cat's lips. Look for recessed, reddened gums and brownish-yellow-green plaque buildup on teeth.
B. Brush a cat's teeth using pet toothpaste and a finger toothbrush two to five times weekly or apply a pet dental hygiene spray with a cotton ball to slow development of dental problems.

III. Veterinary care

A. The cat's teeth should be checked for dental disease at least twice each year by a veterinarian.

B. Treatment or extraction of diseased teeth may be necessary.

INFECTIONS AND FEVER

Infections and fever are unpredictable when left unattended. Many mild infections and fevers may resolve on their own; however, some can be overwhelming and cause long-term complications or death. Even a simple ear infection can be serious.

I. Symptoms of Infections and Fever (some or all may be present)

A. Pain and swelling at site of infection
B. Elevated temperature
C. Listlessness
D. Other general signs of illness such as vomiting, diarrhea, coughing, sneezing, and loss of appetite

II. Home Care

A. Use all medications as prescribed by the veterinarian.
B. Do not deviate from the dosage or the time interval on the label.
C. Use all antibiotics until gone, unless directed otherwise. Sporadic use of antibiotics can cause bacteria to become resistant to treatment.
D. Take the cat's temperature daily to monitor progress. See page 37.

III. Veterinarian Care

A. When you suspect that your cat has an infection, contact your veterinarian immediately; antibiotics may be necessary.

B.   If the cat's condition does not improve, or worsens, while on medication, again contact your veterinarian. It may be necessary to change medications or to perform a culture to further identify the problem.

CANCERS

Certain types of cancers progress slowly and cause only minimal discomfort in their early stages. Cats that have these types of cancers may lead a contented lifestyle for some time. Over time, however, a cat with any cancer is likely to develop complications that may be life-threatening if not tended to promptly. By tending to these problems, you may enable your pet to be comfortable and enjoy a longer life.

A good example of a cancer that typically has a slow progression is feline leukemia. Feline leukemia is incurable, but the symptoms can be eased. For example, if a cat suffers from weight loss or a decrease in appetite from the disease, the cat's diet can be adjusted by your veterinarian to provide more nutrition in smaller quantities.

I. Home Care

A. Loss or decrease in appetite is one of the most common side effects of cancer. Cats can be encouraged to eat by warming their food, hand feeding them, placing their food on a platter instead of in a bowl, and arranging the food in small portions on the platter. If all else fails, try changing the type of food.

B. Avoid stressing pets that have chronic disease.

C. Increase access to water by placing several water bowls throughout the house.

D. Provide more than one litter box for your cat's convenience.

E. Notify your veterinarian of any change in appetite.

F. Keep the cat clean and dry.

G. When a problem arises, contact your veterinarian immediately.

II. Veterinary Care

A. The veterinarian can recommend ways to help keep your cat comfortable.
B. Medications can be used to prevent further complications.
C. A complete physical examination may indicate that surgery may be necessary to prolong the cat's life and provide comfort.
D. Nutritional consultation and diet change may be recommended.

LONG-TERM ILLNESSES

Cats that have chronic diseases, such as liver and kidney disorders, usually cope reasonably well with the problem. Chronic diseases occur gradually, enabling the cat to adjust to the change in organ function without suffering many side effects. With a chronic disease, eventually there will be enough loss in organ function that the cat's condition will begin to decline more quickly.

I. Home Care

A. Loss or decrease in appetite is one of the most common side effects of cancer. Techniques you may use to encourage your cat to eat include warming the cat's food, placing the food on a platter instead of in a bowl, and arranging the food in small portions on the platter rather than in one big clump. If all else fails, try hand feeding or try changing the type of food.

B. Avoid causing stress to pets with chronic disease.

C. Increase access to water by placing several water bowls throughout the house.

D. Provide more than one litter box for the cat's convenience.

E. Notify your veterinarian of any change in appetite or behavior.

F. Keep the cat clean and dry.

G. When a problem arises with a chronically ill cat, contact a veterinarian immediately.

II. Veterinary Care

A. A veterinarian can recommend ways to help keep your cat comfortable.

B. Medications can be used to prevent further deterioration or lessen complications. For example, a potassium deficiency caused by kidney disease is easily treated with a supplement.
C. A complete physical examination may be necessary to determine the best treatment to prolong your cat's life and provide comfort.
D. Nutritional consultation and diet change may be recommended.

SKIN IRRITATIONS

Skin irritations may cause severe discomfort to your pet. In addition, complications can arise from skin conditions, including the spread of infection internally and dehydration (if large areas are affected).

I. Home Care

A. Skin conditions should be tended to immediately to prevent the condition from worsening.
B. Temporary relief can be obtained by bathing your pet in a cat moisturizing shampoo.
C. If your cat is biting and scratching itself, apply a wrap or an Elizabethan collar. (See pages 35 and 47 respectively.)

II. Veterinary Care

A. Untreated skin conditions may lead to serious complications. Medications are available to alleviate skin irritations and hasten healing.
B. Your veterinarian can also determine if your cat's skin condition is one that could be contagious to humans.

SOFT STOOLS/DIARRHEA

Pets can have soft stools or diarrhea without showing other signs of illness. If this condition persists without treatment, the cat could suffer complications, including malnutrition from improper absorption of nutrients, dehydration, and anemia from slow loss of small quantities of blood from bowel irritation.

I.   Home Care

A.   If there is no vomiting, feed the cat 1 teaspoon of Kaopectate® using an eyedropper.

B.   Withhold food for 2-4 hours if diarrhea is present and if there is no other symptom of illness. Withhold both food and water if the cat is also vomiting, but do not withhold water for more than 2 hours. Do not withhold water if the cat is not vomiting. The time period for withholding food should be based on whether your pet is a normal, healthy adult versus a kitten, an elderly cat or a cat with any special or compromising conditions. (If your cat has diabetes or any other type of illness or medical condition, consult your veterinarian first before withholding food and water.) When you do resume feeding your cat, mix cat food (either canned or dry) with an equal amount of water, and make the serving size 1/4 the normal amount of cat food, but feed twice as often. Resume normal feeding within 1/2 to 1 day.

C.   Note the frequency and substance of the diarrhea.

D.   If symptoms persist for more than 4 hours, or if they worsen or return, contact the pet's doctor immediately.

E.   If a cat has other signs along with the diarrhea (e.g., vomiting, loss of coordination, fatigue, etc.) contact a veterinarian.

F.   Because some infections can be transmitted to people, wash your hands after handling the cat or cleaning the litter box.

II. Veterinary Care

A. Your veterinarian may request a stool sample for examination under the microscope (to check for intestinal parasites).
B. Proper diagnosis and medication from your veterinarian can prevent serious side effects from the diarrhea.

INTESTINAL PARASITES

Intestinal parasites, which include worms and protozoa, can cause serious illness if untreated. In general, most infestations are mild at first but then become serious as time progresses. If parasites are left untreated, fatal anemia from chronic blood loss and life-threatening malnutrition can develop. It is important to have a stool sample checked under the microscope for worm eggs. If any eggs are present, your veterinarian can prescribe the proper medication.

The most common parasites in cats include roundworms, tapeworms, hookworms and whipworms. Protozoa infestations include coccidia, giardia and toxoplasmosis. Some of these infections can be spread to people.

I.   Symptoms (some or all may be present)

A.   Weight loss

B.   Diarrhea or soft stools

C.   Blood in stools

D.   Listlessness

E.   Vomiting

F.   Dull hair coat

G.   Pot-bellied appearance

H.   Worms in the stool or under the cat's tail

II.   Home prevention

A.   Change the litter box twice daily (or at a minimum remove the stools twice daily).

B. Wear rubber gloves while cleaning the litter box, and wash your hands afterward; some of these infections can be contagious to people.
C. Practice good flea control. Fleas spread one type of tapeworm.
D. Never feed a cat raw meat.
E. Provide clean, fresh water for your outdoor cat because outside water may contain infectious protozoa or bacteria.
F. If you see any worms in the stool, contact your veterinarian.
G. Avoid over-the-counter worm medications; they may not be the proper choice for your pet's illness.

III. Veterinary care

A. Have a stool specimen examined by a veterinarian twice a year.
B. Use worm medications as directed.

273

EXTERNAL PARASITES - FLEAS

External parasites include fleas, ticks and lice. These parasites not only cause blood loss (sometimes resulting in life-threatening anemia) but may also transmit diseases. Fleas in large numbers can drain enough blood to kill a cat.

I. Symptoms (some or all may be present)

A. Fleas visible crawling through the cat's hair coat or jumping on or off of the cat – They are very small dark insects, so small they are difficult to see. An enlarged illustration appears on page 276.

B. Flea droppings – Even if you cannot see the fleas, you may see flea droppings, which appear as black specks throughout the cat's hair coat. These black specks are actually the fleas' waste products that consist of the cat's blood.

C. Weakness from anemia

D. Weight loss

E. Scratching (though not all cats with fleas will scratch)

II. Pet care

A. Consult your veterinarian. A number of external parasite-control protocols can be prescribed.

B. All products used should be labeled for cats. These products should be used only as directed.

C. If the cat will cooperate, bathe the pet in flea shampoo to remove the fleas and the flea droppings. If not, go to the next step.

D. Treat the cat using a flea spray approved for use on cats. If the cat has received a flea bath (Step C above) then use the flea spray the next day for residual fleas and to keep other fleas off. Treat regularly with flea spray as directed by your veterinarian.

E.   A veterinarian-prescribed flea collar may be used with the spray.

F.   Flea pills are available for your cat, but these pills only prevent mature fleas from reproducing. If your cat has fleas, the flea pills will not kill the fleas.

III. Environmental treatment

A.   Inside the house:
    (1) The cats and the environment should be treated at the same time.
    (2) Vacuum the home thoroughly.
    (3) Discard vacuum cleaner bag.
    (4) Wash the cat's bedding regularly.
    (5) Using hand-held premises spray, treat all corners, baseboards, throw rugs, closets and cracks where foggers will not penetrate. Follow the instructions as directed on the product label.
    (6) Place foggers strategically through the house in each closed room. Foggers will not penetrate through doorways or down hallways. Follow the instructions on the label.
    (7) Check environmental treatment inside the house two weeks after treatment by placing a pan of warm water on the floor before bedtime. Fleas are attracted to warmth and moisture, and if there are any remaining in your house, you should find some in the pan the next day.
    (8) Repeat the above 7 steps in 2-4 weeks, if necessary.

B.   Outside the house treatment:
    (1) Treat the yard with a yard and kennel spray as directed on the product label.
    (2) Keep outside rest areas clean and dry.

IV. Prevention

A. If practical, keep your cat indoors.
B. Do not allow any outside animals indoors.
C. If your cat does venture outside on a regular basis, consider protecting the cat with a flea and tick spray or a flea and tick collar. You may also obtain flea pills for your cat, but these pills do not kill fleas; they only prevent mature fleas from reproducing.
D. Begin flea treatments as soon as you are aware of a flea problem. The longer you wait, the more difficult it will be to get rid of them.

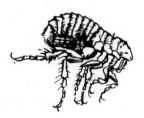

Flea

EXTERNAL PARASITES - LICE

External parasites include fleas, ticks and lice. These parasites not only cause blood loss, sometimes resulting in life-threatening anemia, but may also transmit diseases. Lice in large numbers can drain enough blood to kill a cat.

I. General information

A. Lice are slightly larger than fleas, and unlike fleas, their backs are flat. See illustration below.
B. The eggs or nits are seen as light specks along the hair shafts.

II. Pet care

A. Bathe your cat in a flea and tick shampoo as directed.
B. Once the cat is dry, apply a flea and tick spray approved for use on cats.
C. Contact your family doctor and your veterinarian for details on transmission to people.

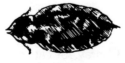

Louse

EXTERNAL PARASITES - TICKS

External parasites include fleas, ticks and lice. These parasites not only cause blood loss, sometimes resulting in life-threatening anemia, but may also transmit diseases. Ticks in large numbers can drain enough blood to kill a cat.

I. General Information

A. Ticks are eight-legged parasites. See illustration on page 279.

B. The tick's body is flat, hard, and shiny but becomes soft and enlarged after feeding on a cat.

C. Ticks may carry diseases such as Lyme disease and Rocky Mountain spotted fever.

D. Ticks embed their mouth parts only into the skin. It is not possible for a tick's head to get left behind in the cat's skin (i.e., when you remove the tick), but it is possible for the area to become infected or irritated mimicking the presence of something under the skin.

II. How to remove a tick

A. Apply a flea and tick spray for cats directly on the tick, and wait one minute. Then, using tweezers or wearing disposable gloves, apply constant pull while grasping the tick's body. The tick should release.

B. Do not try to burn the tick or apply any other type of chemical to the tick. If flea or tick spray is not available, simply pull with constant pressure until the tick releases.
C. Dispose of the tick carefully. Make sure it is dead by spraying the tick or by crushing it, being careful not to touch it with bare hands. The tick can also be flushed down the toilet.
D. Apply antibiotic ointment to the area where the tick was removed.
E. If any unusual symptoms develop after the removal of the tick, contact your veterinarian.

IV. Prevention

A. If practical, keep your cat indoors.
B. Do not allow any outside animals indoors.
C. If your cat does venture outside on a regular basis, consider using a tick spray or a flea and tick collar on the pet.

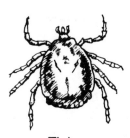

Tick

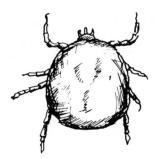

Engorged Tick

PART 8

MISCELLANEOUS

DELIVERIES

While most deliveries are routine and can be accomplished without any human intervention, sometimes complications occur. This chapter will assist you in identifying delivery problems.

I. Preparation for Delivery

A. Gather the following materials: a large box, clean towels, thread, warm water bottles and emergency formula. (See page 286 for a homemade emergency formula.)

B. Make sure the cat has a clean nesting area for the delivery. A box 2 feet square and 6 inches high lined with a clean towel is ideal.

C. Handle the cat as little as possible.

II. Helping with a Delivery

A. Try not to disturb the cat during the delivery process, but try to monitor her progress by quietly observing her actions.

B. If a kitten is being passed and is having difficulty clearing the vulva, you may exert gentle downward pressure on the kitten to help it pass.

C. If the mother is not cleaning the kittens after delivery, use a towel and remove any fluid from the nose and mouth. Then dry the kitten using a gentle rubbing action.

D. Occasionally the umbilical cord will not separate from the mother and kitten. If this occurs, take a thread and tie a knot 1/2 inch from the kitten's belly, and then cut the cord with scissors between the knot and the mother cat. This will prevent bleeding from tearing the cord. (See illustration on page 284.)

E. If a kitten is not breathing, continue to stimulate the kitten by rubbing it vigorously; at the same time blow into its nose every 5 seconds to give it air. Try this for at least 5 minutes.

F. The kittens should be placed at the mother's breast to ensure they nurse. Keep track of any kittens that do not nurse; they may need to be hand fed.

G. If the kittens cry, they may be hungry, cold, or sick. Contact your veterinarian if the crying persists.

III. Signs of a Difficult Delivery

A. If more than 20 minutes pass between kittens and the mother is having strong contractions, call your veterinarian.

B. If labor continues for more than an hour without the birth of a kitten, call your veterinarian.

C. When there is a weak contraction for a period of 1 hour between bouts of active labor, but no kitten is delivered, call your veterinarian.

D. If you observe any evidence of unusual pain during the delivery, such as crying or excessive biting or licking of the hind quarters, call your veterinarian.

E. If the pregnancy exceeds 70 days, call your veterinarian.

F. If there is an unusual discharge coming from the vulva under the tail, call your veterinarian. Normal discharge is green (not black, bloody, cloudy, or foul-smelling).

G. If there is normal greenish discharge without the birth of a kitten, call your veterinarian.

H. If the cat shows symptoms of illness, like depression, vomiting, diarrhea or weakness, call your veterinarian.

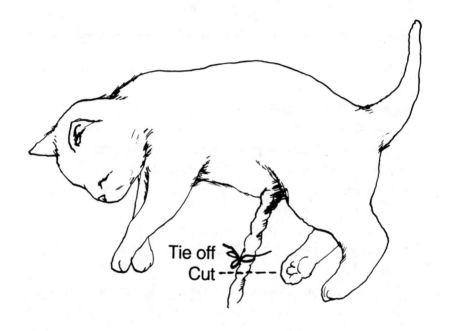

Tie off
Cut

RAISING ORPHAN KITTENS

When kittens have been abandoned or when the mother does not nurse her kittens, the kittens will need special care if they are to survive. Raising orphan kittens can be very rewarding but demands much time, motivation, and devotion. Unlike adult cats, kittens have little body reserve and need highly regimented feeding and care schedules.

I. Materials Needed

A. Cotton balls
B. Light bulb or heat lamp
C. Pet nurser
D. Eyedropper
E. Formula
F. Scale for weighing
G. Thermometer

II. Hygiene/Husbandry

A. The kitten's nest area should be cleaned three times daily to prevent disease. Bed the area with newspaper or towels.

B. Store all formula as directed on the label to prevent spoilage.

C. Chilling is one of the leading causes of death among newborns. Keep the kittens warm with a heat lamp, heating pad, or hot water bottles. However, take care that the heat source is not too hot, and prepare a box that provides enough room for the kittens to move away from the heat source if they become too hot. Heating pads must be monitored closely to regulate temperature and prevent fire hazard. **Do not place a heating pad or hot water bottle on top of the kittens.**

D. The environmental temperature should be kept at 85-90 degrees from days 1-7. The temperature should be lowered to 80 degrees during week 2. Weeks 3-5, the temperature should be lowered to 75 degrees, then decreased again to 70 degrees at week 6.

E. Urinations and bowel movements must be stimulated after each meal. This is accomplished by moistening a cotton ball with warm water and gently wiping the kitten's bottom and abdomen.

F. Weigh each kitten and take its temperature daily.

III. Feeding

A. Use a pet nurser, if available, to feed the kittens. The hole in the nurser should leak milk slowly from the bottle without pressure. An eyedropper may be used temporarily if a nurser is unavailable.

B. Never feed a chilled kitten; make sure the orphan is warm prior to feeding.

C. Commercial formulas for newborns or infants are recommended over homemade diets. Homemade diets tend to lack balanced nutrition. If a commercial formula is not available, the following can be substituted:

EMERGENCY FORMULA RECIPE #1
8 oz. homogenized whole milk
1 teaspoon salad oil
2 egg yolks
1 drop infant vitamins

EMERGENCY FORMULA RECIPE #2
1/3 cup nonfat dried milk
1/4 cup cottage cheese
1/8 cup corn oil
Add enough water to make 2 cups volume
Mix in blender

D. When using a commercially-available formula, follow the directions on the label regarding preparation, the frequency of feedings, and the amount to be fed.

E. When using homemade formula or some prepared formulas, follow these guidelines:

    (1) In the first week of the cat's life – 2 teaspoons every 4 hours.

    (2) In the second week – 2 1/2 teaspoons every 4 hours.

    (3) In the third week – 3 teaspoons every 6 hours.

    (4) In the fourth week – 4 teaspoons every 6 hours. During this week, begin to mix the formula with canned kitten food. Offer these meals on a flat plate and allow the kitten to play in the mixture to encourage self feeding.

F. Urinations and bowel movements must be stimulated after each meal. This is accomplished by moistening a cotton ball with warm water and gently wiping the kitten's bottom and abdomen.

G. Overfeeding may cause diarrhea. Consult a veterinarian immediately if diarrhea occurs because kittens dehydrate easily.

IV. Signs of Illness

A. Crying (indicates that the kittens are either hungry, chilled, or sick)

B. Restlessness

C. Loss of appetite

D. Fever

E. Weight loss or lack of weight gain

F. Pot-bellied appearance

G. Vomiting or diarrhea

FALSE EMERGENCIES

Because cats lack the ability to communicate the exact nature of their problems, some events can be misinterpreted as emergencies. Heat periods and hairballs are two situations that may seem like emergencies, but they are not cause for alarm. However, they do need to be understood and addressed appropriately.

Female cats reach sexual maturity and begin to go into heat between 5-12 months of age. Female cats often exhibit a marked behavioral change during their heat periods.

The vomiting of hairballs is a common phenomenon in cats. The retching prior to vomiting can appear quite violent, but it is not dangerous to the cat. Vomiting is the cat's natural response to removing the accumulation of hair from the stomach. If the hair is not passed through the digestive tract and is not vomited, then the situation can turn into an emergency; the hairball may get so large in the stomach that food will not be able to pass through the cat's system.

I. Heat Periods

A. When a cat is in heat, it may exhibit a variety of unusual behavior, including:
  (1) Rolling on the floor
  (2) Squirming and stretching with its tail and hindquarters raised off the floor
  (3) Purring or meowing loudly.
B. Some cats may experience a decrease in appetite during the heat period.
C. If there is doubt about the cause of the cat's behavioral change, consult a veterinarian.
D. Unless your cat is going to be used for breeding, you should

have her spayed. The reasons for having your female cat spayed include:

(1) The spayed cat will cease having heat periods.
(2) Spayed cats have a lower incidence of breast cancer and fatal infections of the uterus.
(3) Pregnancy exposes cats to unnecessary health risks.
(4) There is an overpopulation of cats; unwanted pregnancies contribute to this number.

II. Hairballs

A. Hairball preventive preparations, a beef-flavored gel, can be purchased from the cat's veterinarian. Instructions should be followed on the back of the container.

B. Most cats like the gel and will often take it as a treat, but for those who do not like the taste, the gel can be mixed with a small amount of food, wiped on the cat's paws or applied directly into the cat's mouth.

C. Vaseline® (petroleum jelly) and mineral oil should be avoided because they are tasteless, can cause choking, and can be aspirated into the lungs.

D. If the hairball problem persists even after treatment, or if other symptoms of illness are present, consult the cat's doctor.

THE HOSPITALIZED CAT

When your pet must be hospitalized, you should make a list of questions for your veterinarian. In this chapter, a list of questions has been compiled for you, though you may wish to add more depending on the situation. If your cat does need hospitalization, don't simply ask the questions, but also write down the answers. If you make a written record of the answers, you will be better able to track your cat's progress based on the initial observations of the veterinarian.

I. Basic Guidelines

A. Leave a telephone number where someone can be reached at all times so that any changes in the cat's condition or treatment can be discussed.
B. Check with the doctors about their pet visitation policy. Visitation is helpful not only to the pet but also for the owner.
C. If financial limits are affecting the care your cat may receive, inquire whether financial aid is available.
D. Determine how many progress reports will be shared during the day and whether you should call or they should call you.

II. Questions To Ask About the Problem

A. What is my cat's problem?
B. Does my pet have more than one problem, and, if so, are the problems related?
C. If there are several possible problems, are there tests to confirm the diagnosis?

III. Questions to Ask About Determining the Problem (Diagnosis)

A. What tests are available to diagnose my pet?
B. What information will the tests give?
C. Can the test results change the type of treatment my cat is receiving?
D. What is the cost of testing?
E. How invasive are the tests? How much pain will they cause and is there any risk associated with the tests?

IV. Questions To Ask About the Outcome (Prognosis)

A. What is my cat's prognosis?
B. Will this condition return?
C. Will this condition have any long-term side effects?
D. What is an average recovery time?

V. Questions To Ask About the Treatment

A. What will the treatment involve?
B. How much time will treatments take?
C. How expensive are the medications?
D. What side effects will be involved with the medicines?
E. If surgery is recommended:
　　(1) Is there more than one procedure that can be done?
　　(2) Is there a medical alternative to a surgical procedure?
　　(3) How many of these surgeries do you perform per year?
　　(4) Should I see a specialist?
F. What type of care will need to be provided after the cat returns home?
G. Are follow-up doctor visits recommended?

THE LOST CAT

One of the most frightening events for a cat owner is to lose a pet. Because of a cat's curiosity and instinct, it is often prone to roam. In particular, unaltered cats have a high incidence of roaming because of urges to find a mate. Proper identification will improve your chances of recovering your lost cat. If your initial attempts to locate your pet are unsuccessful, do not give up hope; many animals return home days, weeks, or months later. Even with proper identification, the cat's chances of being found can be greatly increased by following the steps described below.

I. Information about the Lost Cat

A. List the cat's sex, breed, color, age, name and any distinguishing characteristics.
B. Make a list of several numbers (including the veterinarian's number) for people to call if the cat is found.
C. Find a picture of the cat, if possible.
D. Decide whether to offer a reward, and if so, what amount.

II. Daily Cat-Owner Efforts

A. Visit shelters daily to search for the cat.
   (Do not assume someone will call if the pet arrives at the shelter. Most shelters deal with hundreds of pets each day. Daily visits are important because cats are frequently euthanized after two days if not claimed or adopted.)
B. Contact all local veterinarians by phone about the missing cat.

C. Drive through local neighborhoods calling for and asking about the cat.

D. Have neighbors help in the search. Ask them to check their garages and storage sheds.

E. Post "Lost Cat" notices. See Appendix page 296.
   (1) Include all identifying information. (See Section I above.)
   (2) Include a picture.
   (3) Indicate if there is a reward.
   (4) Use waterproof ink and sturdy paper or poster board.
   (5) Make the sign large so that it can be read from a distance.
   (6) Post signs at all major intersections within at least a 3-mile radius of the cat's home.
   (7) Post signs at local pet stores and other businesses (with their permission).
   (8) Post signs at veterinary offices.

III. Organizations to Contact

A. Contact the local humane society.
   (1) Ask whether they have your pet.
   (2) Inquire about volunteers who run a lost and found or rescue service.

B. Contact other local shelters such as the dog/animal pound.

IV. Use of the Media

A. Run a classified advertisement for at least two weeks.

B. Check with radio and television; they often donate time during their news broadcasts to help find lost pets.

APPENDICES

LOST PET INFORMATION

Use the following form to help find a lost cat. Duplicate this form and post it according to the instructions found in the chapter The Lost Cat (starting on page 292).

LOST CAT

DESCRIPTION/BREED_____

COLOR(S)_____

SEX _____ AGE_____ WEIGHT_____ HEIGHT_____

COAT LENGTH _____

IDENTIFYING MARKS_____

TYPE AND COLOR OF COLLAR _____

LICENSE#_____ RABIES TAG#_____

AREA LOST _____

DATE LOST _____

CAT'S NAME_____

OWNER'S NAME _____

ADDRESS _____

HOME PHONE_____ WORK PHONE_____

ATTACH PICTURE HERE

MEDICAL HEALTH RECORD

Owner's Name _____

Address _____

_____

Home Phone_____ Work Phone_____

Friend/Family For Emergency Contact _____

_____

Cat's Name _____

Breed_____

Date of Birth _____

Special Diet _____

Date	Vaccination Type
_____	_____
_____	_____
_____	_____
_____	_____
_____	_____
_____	_____
_____	_____
_____	_____
_____	_____
_____	_____
_____	_____

Date	Stool Examinations & Treatment
_____	_____
_____	_____
_____	_____
_____	_____

297

Date	Medical Examination/Treatment/Weight
_____	_____
_____	_____
_____	_____
_____	_____
_____	_____
_____	_____

Emergency Numbers
    Veterinarian_____
    After-Hour Veterinarian_____
    Poison Control_____
    National Animal Poison Control Center_____
    Fire Department_____

EMERGENCY WORKSHEET

Temperature _____ Pulse _____ Respirations _____

Where is the major problem located?
        ___ mouth
        ___ eyes
        ___ neck
        ___ chest (heart and lungs)
        ___ abdomen
        ___ back
        ___ urinary tract
        ___ legs
        ___ skin
        ___ nervous system

What kind of symptoms or problems are present? List them.

_____

_____

_____

_____

How long have the symptoms been present?
        _____ minutes _____ hours _____ days _____ weeks

Are the symptoms becoming _____ better _____ worse _____ same?

Have these problems occurred before?

Does the cat appear to be
        ___ depressed
        ___ disoriented
        ___ in pain
        ___ incoherent
        ___ excitable

NORMAL VITAL SIGNS FOR CATS

Temperature   100.5 to 102.5 degrees Fahrenheit

Pulse/Heart Rate   110 to 140 beats per minute

Respiratory Rate   24 to 28 breaths per minute

The above signs are for a normal mature cat at rest. An excited cat, or one that has been running around, will have an elevated heart rate and an elevated respiratory rate. However, elevated vital signs for a cat at rest may be a sign of infection, disease, overheating or a variety of other health problems. Low vital signs may indicate that the cat is in shock. See Problem/Condition - Shock.

PREVENTIVE HEALTH CARE

Good health care is paramount in disease prevention. The old saying "an ounce of prevention is worth a pound of cure" definitely applies to cats. Many fatal infections can be prevented by proper health care in the form of vaccinations, dental care, and regular worm examinations. Other advances in feline medicine, some in the form of blood tests, can also be utilized to extend a cat's lifespan.

I. Feline Leukemia and Feline Immunosuppressive Virus Testing

A. Feline leukemia and feline immunosuppressive virus (FIV) are both viruses that are contagious among cats but are not contagious to people. At present, there is a vaccination for feline leukemia, but there is no vaccination for FIV.

B. All cats should be tested for the diseases to protect healthy cats from those that test positive for the diseases. Cats that test positive for FIV should be isolated from those that do not have the virus.

C. Cats that test negative for feline leukemia should be vaccinated against the disease, especially if they venture outdoors where they may be exposed to other cats. Having your cat vaccinated against feline leukemia is extremely important because there is no known cure for the disease.

D. A cat with either of these diseases can experience any of three disease processes:

  (1) The cat can be a carrier of the disease but not be ill.

  (2) The cat may become ill from the disease but respond to medicines to ease the symptoms. (Note: There is no cure for either of these diseases.)

  (3) The cat may become ill and die from the virus. If a cat becomes ill from either of the diseases, the cat may develop

301

cancers, reproductive problems and/or immune
complications.

E. Cats that test positive sometimes are prone to developing other
diseases and may have slow recovery from illnesses in general.

II. Infections that Vaccinations Prevent

A. Vaccinations are important to prevent many serious infections, as
well as to decrease the severity of an infection if one occurs.

B. Diseases that can be prevented by vaccinations include feline
rhinotracheitis, chlamydia, calici virus, feline leukemia, feline
infectious peritonitis (FIP), panleukopenia (feline distemper) and
rabies. The first three diseases are upper-respiratory infections.
Feline leukemia is an incurable disease that causes a host of
disorders including various cancers. Feline infectious peritonitis
is a fatal disease that causes inflammation of the blood vessels
leading to peritonitis (inflammation of the abdominal wall),
seizures, eye disorders, diarrhea, difficulty breathing and a
swollen abdomen. Panleukopenia causes symptoms of vomiting
and diarrhea and is often fatal. Rabies, an almost universally
fatal disease, is carried by a variety of animals and can be
transmitted to people.

III. Kitten Vaccinations and Care

A. Kittens without vaccinations have very little immunity to fight
infections, especially after they are weaned from their mother.

B. Vaccinations are important to prevent many serious infections, as
well as to decrease the severity of an infection if one occurs.

C. Kittens should start vaccinations for rhinotracheitis, calici virus,

chlamydia (three upper-respiratory infections) and
panleukopenia (distemper) at 6 weeks of age.

D. Kittens should receive booster vaccinations for these diseases
at ages 9 weeks, 12 weeks and 15 weeks. The booster
vaccinations are important because the kittens need a series of
shots to provide them with adequate immunity to protect them
for 1 year.

E. After feline leukemia and feline immunosuppressive virus
testing at 10 weeks of age, the kittens may begin their
vaccinations against feline leukemia. They will need
2 vaccinations at 3-week intervals in order to protect them for
1 year.

F. Also at 10 weeks of age the kitten may start protective
vaccinations against feline infectious peritonitis. This
vaccination is administered by nose drops rather than injection.
The kittens will need 2 sets of nose drops 3 weeks apart to
provide 1 year of immunity.

G. At 3 to 4 month of age, kittens should be vaccinated against
rabies. The vaccination will protect against the disease for 1 year
or 3 years depending upon the vaccine.

H. Some veterinarians recommend vaccinations for all the above
diseases. Others recommend feline leukemia and feline
infectious peritonitis only for those cats that are at high risk
(i.e., outdoor pets). In general, it is advisable to give your cat
a complete set of vaccinations if the pet is likely to come into
contact with any other cats. Consult your veterinarian for more
information about vaccination schedules.

IV. Elective Surgery – Spaying/Neutering

A. Neutering helps prevent prostatic cancer and enlargement in
male cats.

B. Neutering prevents testicular cancer in male cats.

C. Neutering generally improves your cat's temperament.

D. Neutering helps prevent the marking of territory with urine.

E. Altering male and female cats will decrease roaming and running away.

F. Altering cats prevents unwanted cat pregnancies.

G. In female cats, the incidence of breast cancer may be decreased by having the cat spayed.

H. Both male and female cats can usually have surgery as early as 5-6 months of age. Consult your veterinarian for additional information.

V. Adult Vaccinations and Care

A. All adults not tested for feline leukemia and feline immunosuppressive virus should have blood analyzed for the diseases.

B. Adults not vaccinated as kittens need two vaccinations for all diseases with 3 weeks between shots, except for rabies. Rabies vaccination requires only one starting vaccine with routine booster shots every year to every 3 years.

C. Adults vaccinated as kittens need vaccination boosters every year. Rabies vaccinations may be good for 3 years depending on the type. Check with the cat's doctor.

D. Once per year a veterinarian should check a fecal (bowel movement) specimen under the microscope for worm eggs or other microscopic parasites.

E. A complete physical examination every year is advisable.

PHYSICAL EXAMINATION

The key to early detection of disease and health problems is knowing what to look for and how to look for it. A standard physical examination is a primary tool used by all veterinarians both to identify difficulties and to evaluate the seriousness of an emergency. By becoming familiar with the content of a physical examination, you will be able to understand your cat's symptoms better, and you will be better able to provide relevant information about your cat to your veterinarian.

I. History

As a first step in performing a physical examination, the veterinarian will ask you about the past activities of your cat. Veterinarians refer to this as a pet's history. A history helps identify numerous potential problems. For example, did the pet just return from being outside, or did a family member just treat the cat for fleas, or has the cat been urinating outside the litter box?

II. Subjective Observations (Attitude)

Next, the veterinarian will note the general attitude of the cat. Is the cat excited or depressed? Has the cat's activity level increased or decreased? Does the cat seem to be alert? Is there anything unusual about the cat's attitude or behavior?

III. Objective Observations (Physical Signs)

After the veterinarian has observed the pet's general attitude, he or she will start looking for symptoms (i.e., perform objective observations) to help pinpoint illness. The two methods veterinarians use to perform objective observations are the body system review and the spatial arrangement review.

The body system review consists of evaluating the pet's health according to the different functions of the body. The body systems include the digestive tract, urogenital system (urinary and reproductive tracts), nervous system, integument system (skin), musculoskeletal system (muscle and bone), reproductive system, cardiopulmonary system (heart and lungs) and the special senses (sight, hearing and smell).

The spatial system starts at the nose and ends at the tail. The veterinarian examines the cat's entire body looking at any and all organs, muscles, bones, etc. one body part at a time (e.g., head, chest, hind quarters). Some veterinarians use a combination of the body system and the spatial arrangement.

IV. Health Checklist/Inventory

Refer to the following tables as checklists you might use to provide information to your veterinarian concerning the health of your cat. These are the types of checklists your veterinarian will use to evaluate your pet.

A. Eyes, Ears, Nose and Throat Checklist

_____ Are the eyes clear? Cloudy? Red?
_____ Is there discharge coming from the eyes?
_____ Is the cat rubbing its eyes?
_____ Are both eyes affected?

306

____ Is one eye bigger than the other?

____ Are the eyes moving back and forth when the cat is at rest?

____ Is the head tilted?

____ Is there any discharge coming from the ears?

____ Are the ear flaps swollen?

____ Is there discharge coming from the nose?

____ If there is nasal discharge, is it from both nostrils?

____ If there is nasal discharge, is it bloody, clear, or cloudy?

____ Are the gums pink? If not, what color are they? Blue? White?

____ Are there diseased teeth in the mouth?

____ Is the cat pawing at its mouth?

____ Is the cat drooling?

____ Is there blood in the cat's mouth?

B.   Heart and Lungs (Cardiopulmonary) Checklist

Symptoms that may denote problems with the heart and lungs include coughing, difficult breathing, panting, fainting, collapse, blue gums, enlarged abdomen, and wheezing. Some emergency situations involving the cardiopulmonary system include heart failure, asthma, trauma (physical injury), infections and cancers. It is interesting to note that sneezing is usually associated with upper respiratory illness whereas coughing is usually associated with lower respiratory tract disorders. If you identify any of these problems, answer the following questions:

____ Is the cat coughing? Is the cough dry or productive (i.e., producing mucus)?

____ Is the cat having difficulty breathing? Does the cat's abdomen move and heave when the pet breathes?

____ Does the cat's abdomen appear enlarged?

____ Has the cat fainted or collapsed?

____ Is the cat wheezing?

____ How long have the symptoms been present?

____ How long do these spells last?

C.   Digestive Tract Checklist

Your cat's appetite should be monitored. Cats that have food available 24 hours per day pose a challenge because it is difficult to ascertain when and how much they are eating. If you feed your cat at specified times and remove any uneaten food between meals, it will be easier to monitor your cat's appetite.

Make sure your cat is fed at least twice per day. Some cats with sensitive stomachs may need to have food available on a continuous basis, but in that case it may be possible to monitor their appetite by having dry food always available but providing canned food only once or twice per day.

Digestive symptoms include vomiting, diarrhea, painful abdomen, distended abdomen, constipation, loss of appetite, and increased digestive noises. Common digestive tract problems include food poisoning, pancreatitis, cancers, foreign objects, toxins, parasites, electrolyte imbalances, kidney disease and liver disease. To help identify any of these problems, answer the following questions:

___ Has the cat been vomiting? If so, does the food look digested?

___ Is the pet eating? Has its appetite increased or decreased?

___ Is the cat eating only favorite foods?

___ How long has it been since the last meal?

___ Are the bowel movements normal? Soft? Watery? Dry?

___ Is there mucous or blood present in the cat's stool?

___ Are the cat's stools black or clay colored?

___ Is the cat constipated? How long has it been since the last bowel movement?

D.   Urinary and Reproductive Tract Checklist

The most serious urinary tract problem is blockage. When a cat changes its litter-box behavior (i.e., does not urinate at all or urinates outside the box), it is important to rule out medical causes before blaming the cat for a behavioral problem. Early symptoms of blockage include straining in the litter box, urinating outside the litter box, crying while trying to urinate, lying in the litter box and severe depression. Frequent urinations and blood in the urine may also be signs of an impending medical emergency. Common reproductive and urinary tract problems include cystitis (inflamed bladder), urinary tract blockage, uterus infections, bladder stones, ruptured bladder from trauma, kidney disease and cancers. To help identify any of these problems, answer the following questions:

___ Is the cat urinating more frequently or less frequently?

___ Is the cat straining in the litter box?

___ Is the cat urinating outside the litter box?

___ Does the cat cry when trying to urinate?

___ Is the cat lying in the litter box?

___ Is the cat urinating less volume or more volume than usual?

___ Is the cat drinking more water than usual?

___ Is the cat persistently licking its genital area?

___ Is there any discharge coming from the cat's genital area?

E.   Integument (Skin) Checklist

Skin problems can arise from a multitude of causes including external parasites, burns, frostbite, lacerations and abrasions, allergies, nervous/emotional disorders and growths (benign or malignant). To help identify any skin difficulties, use the following checklist:

___ Are there any hairless areas on the cat? If so, are these areas irritated?

___ Is the cat scratching continuously?

___ Are there any lumps on the skin? If so, what size?

___ Are there any punctures or lacerations?

___ Is there any evidence of fleas or other external parasites?

___ Is there any evidence of a rash anywhere on the cat's body? If so, where is the rash?

F. Musculoskeletal (Muscle and Bone) & Nervous System Checklist

Some emergencies involving these systems include trauma, fractures, torn ligaments, disc disease, vestibular (inner ear) problems, and infections.

___ Can the cat move?
___ Is the cat limping? If so, which leg?
___ Is the cat stumbling?
___ Is the cat dragging its legs?
___ Is the cat mentally alert?
___ Does the cat walk in circles?
___ Is the cat uncoordinated?

BIBLIOGRAPHY

Alber, John I., and Delores M. Alber. *Baby-Safe Houseplants & Cut Flowers.* Highland, IL: Genus Books, 1991.

Arthurs, Kathryn, ed. *How to Grow House Plants.* 2nd ed. Menlo Park: Lane Publishing, 1974.

Fenner, William R., D.V.M., ed. *Quick Reference to Veterinary Medicine.* 2nd ed. Philadelphia: J. P. Lippincott, 1991.

Florists' Transworld Delivery Association. *Professional Guide to Green Plants.* Florists' Transworld Delivery Association, 1976.

Fowler, Murray E., D.V.M. *Plant Poisoning in Small Companion Animals.* St. Louis: Ralston Purina, 1981.

Fraser, Clarence M., ed. *The Merck Veterinary Manual.* 6th, 7th eds. Rathway, NJ: Merck & Co., 1986, 1991.

Holzworth, Jean, D.V.M. *Diseases of the Cat: Medicine and Surgery.* Philadelphia: W. B. Saunders, 1987.

Hoskins, Johnny D. *Veterinary Pediatrics: Dogs and Cats from Birth to Six Months.* Philadelphia: W. B. Saunders, 1990.

Kirk, Robert W., D.V.M., and Stephen I. Bister, D.V.M. *Handbook of Veterinary Procedures and Emergency Treatment.* 4th ed. Philadelphia: W. B. Saunders, 1985.

Levy, Charles Kingsley, and Richard B. Primack. *A Field Guide to Poisonous Plants and Mushrooms of North America.* Brattleboro, VT: The Stephen Greene Press, 1984.

National Animal Poison Control Center. *Household Plant List.* Urbana: University of Illinois College of Veterinary Medicine.

Osweiler, Gary D., D.V. M., Thomas L. Carson, D.V.M., William B. Buck, D.V.M., and Gary A. VanGelder, D.V.M. *Clinical and Diagnostic Veterinary Toxicology.* 3rd ed. Dubuque, IA: Kendell/Hunt, 1985.

Random House Webster's College Dictionary. New York: Random House, 1991.

Sherding, Robert G., D.V.M., ed. *The Cat: Diseases and Clinical Management.* 2nd ed. Livingstone, NY: Churchill, 1994.

Taylor, Norman. *Taylor's Guide to Perennials.* Ed. Gordon P. DeWolf. Boston: Houghton Mifflin, 1961.

Tuckington, Carol. *The Home Health Guide to Poisons and Antidotes.* New York: Facts on File, 1994.

Woodward, Lucia. *Poisonous Plants: A Color Field Guide.* New York: Hippocrene Books, 1985.

INDEX

Abdomen
  painful, 79, 81, 129, 131
    See poisonous plants, 182-231
  protruding, 103
Abrasions, 53
  and bleeding, 134-135
Abrasive cleaners, 236
Abscess, bite wound, 54-55, 136-137
Accident-proofing your home, 9-11
Acetaminophen, 56-57, 234-235
Acids, 236-237
Adhesives, 178. *See* poisoning
  general procedures, 176-177
Adult cat, vaccinations, 304
Advil®. *See* ibuprofin, 97, 248
Airway, blocked. *See* choking, 73-75,
  illus. 75, 145-147
Alkalis, 236-237
Allergies, 58
  and bumps, 144
  and eyes, 157
  and plants, 232
  and scratching, 166-167
Alocasia, 183
Aloe vera, 183
Amaryllis, 183
Ammonia, 236
Amphetamines, 178. *See* poisoning
  general procedures, 176-177
Anemia, 60
  and aspirin toxicity, 63, 242
  and soft stools/diarrhea, 270
Animal shelters and lost cat, 292
Ant
  bites, 119-120
  ingestion of. *See* insect
    ingestion, 100
Antidandruff shampoo, 178. *See*

poisoning general procedures,
  176-177
Antidepressants, 178. *See* poisoning
  general procedures, 176-177
Antidotes to poisons. *See* specific
  poisons, 234-258
  poisonous plants, 182-231
Antifreeze, 61-62, 238-239
Antihistamines, 178. *See* poisoning
  general procedures, 176-177
Antipsychotics, 178. *See* poisoning
  general procedures, 176-177
Antiseptics
  and wound care, 33-34
  as poison, 236
Anxiety and choking, 73
Appetite, loss of
  and abscesses, 54
  and anemia, 60
  and cancer, 265
  and digestive upset, 81
  and infections, 263
  and uterus infection, 129
  and vomiting, 131
  and yard chemicals, 132
Apple, 184
Apprehensiveness and strychnine
  poisoning, 121, 256
Aquarium products, 236
Arrhythmia, 71
Arsenic, 240
Asparagus fern, 231
Asphyxiation
  See carbon monoxide, 113, 178
  See choking, 73-75, *illus. 75,*
    145-147
  See poisonous plants, 182-231
  See smoke inhalation, 113-115

313

Aspiration of fluid, 145
Aspirin, 63-64, 242-243
Asthma, 142
Atropine, 178. *See* poisoning general
procedures, 176-177
Automobile batteries, 236
Autumn crocus, 184
Azalea, 185

Balance, loss of, 163
Barbiturates, 178. *See* poisoning
general procedures, 176-177
Batteries
automobile, 236
small household, 236
Bee
ingestion of. *See* insect
ingestion, 100
stings, 65
Beetles, ingestion of. *See* insect
ingestion, 100
Behavioral changes
affecting restraint, 20-21
and depression, 172
and lead poisoning, 249
and urinary-tract blockage, 127
See also anxiety,
apprehensiveness, loss of
appetite
Belly
pot, 272, 287
upset. *See* vomiting, 131
See also abdomen
Benzodiazepines, 178. *See* poisoning
general procedures, 176-177
Bird-of-paradise, 185
Birth defects in offspring and
poisonous plant ingestion,
194, 201, 207, 212
Birth of kittens, 282
Bite marks, 66
snake, 117
Bite wound abscess, 54-55, 136-137

Bite wounds
general, 54-55, 66, 136-137
snake, 117
spider, 119
Black locust, 185
Black widow spider, 119
Bladder control, loss of, 107
Bleach, 178, 236
Bleeding
abrasions, 134
bite wound abscess, 136
control of, 31-32
external, 67-68
gunshot wounds, 138
internal, 67-68, 105, 195
lacerations, 134
trauma in general, 140
Bleeding control, 31-32
See also abrasions, bite wound
abscess, fractures, gunshot
wounds, lacerations
Bleeding-heart, 186
Blindness
and finger cherry ingestion, 202
and seizures, 107
See eye emergencies, 83
Blocked airway. *See* choking, 73-75,
illus. 75, 145-147
Blood
accumulating under skin, 67
and pus, 54, 136
bleeding control, 31-32
in feces, 76, 191, 253, 272
in urine, 67, 119, 216, 253
spurting, 31
See also bleeding
Borates, 178. *See* poisoning general
procedures, 176-177
Boxwood, 186
Bowel control, loss of, 107
See litter box habits, 161-162
Bowel movement
and protruding rectum, 103

314

lack of, 78
Bowels, exposed, 103
Breathing
    difficulties, 142-143
    normal respiration, 300
    See also poisonous plants
Broad bean. *See* fava bean, 201
Bromethalin, 178. *See* poisoning
    general procedures, 176-177
Brown recluse spider, 119
Bruises
    and lameness, 159
    and cycad plants, 195
    and rat poison, 105
Buckeye, 187
Buddhist pine, 187
Bugs, ingestion of. *See* insect
    ingestion, 100
Bumble bees. *See* bee stings, 65
Bumps, 144
Burns, 70-71
    acid, 71, 237
    alkali, 71, 237
    chemical, 71
Buttercup, 188
Butterfly, ingestion of. *See* insect
    ingestion, 100
Buttons, ingestion of. *See* choking,
    73

Caladium, 188
Calamondin orange, 188
Calcium oxalate crystals, 188, 189,
    192, 198, 199
Calici virus, 302
Calla lily, 189
Camphor, 178. *See* poisoning
    general procedures, 176-177
Cancers, 265
Carbolic acid, 236
Carbon monoxide, 113, 178
Cardiopulmonary resuscitation
    (CPR), 40-43, *illus. 41,43*

See also heart disease, heat stroke,
    lung disease, poison, seizures,
    shock
Castor bean, 190
Cat box. *See* litter box habits, 161-
    162
Cat-proofing your home, 9-11
Ceriman. *See* philodendron, 220
Charming dieffenbachia. *See* dumb
    cane, 198
Checklist, health, 306-310
Chemical burns, 71
Cherry, 190
Chilling, 95
Chlamydia, 302
Chlorinated hydrocarbons, 178. *See*
    poisoning general procedures,
    176-177
Chocolate, 72, 244
Choking, 73-75, *illus. 75*, 145-147
Cholecalciferol, 178. *See* poisoning
    general procedures, 176-177
Christmas plants
    holly, 205
    mistletoe, 215
    poinsettia, 221, 231
Christmas rose, 191
Christmas tree tinsel, 9, 11
Chrysanthemum, 191, 231
Cicada, ingestion of. *See* insect
    ingestion, 100
Cineraria, 192
Claw, torn. *See* torn toenail, 125
Cleaning solutions, 236
Cleansing of wound, 33
Coal tar, 178. *See* poisoning general
    procedures, 176-177
Cocaine, 178. *See* poisoning general
    procedures, 176-177
Coccidia, 272
Cockroach, ingestion of. *See* insect
    ingestion, 100
Colitis, 76-77

Collapse, 148-150
Collar
  Elizabethan, 47-49
  regular, 8
Colocasia. *See* elephant's ear, 199
Consciousness, loss of
  and collapse, 148
  and heart disease, 89
Coma
  and collapse, 148
  and hypothermia, 95
  and smoke inhalation, 113
  and snake bites, 117
  See also poisonous plants
Confusion
  and hypothermia, 95
  and inner ear disease, 99
  and seizures, 107
Constipation, 78
Constricted pupils and plant
  ingestion, 206, 216
Convulsions
  and seizures, 107
  and snail bait poisoning, 116
Coordination, loss of, 163
Cordatum, 192
Corn plant, 193
Cornstalk plant, 193
Corydalis, 193
Coughing, 151
  See choking, 73
CPR, 40-43, *illus. 41, 43*
Creosote, 178. *See* poisoning general
  procedures, 176-177
Crotalaria, 194
Croton, 194
Crowfoot family. *See* buttercup, 188
Crown of thorns, 195
Cuban laurel, 195
Cuticle remover, 236
Cuts. *See* lacerations, 134
Cycad, 195
Cyanide, 178, 184, 190, 205

Cyclamen, 196
Cysts, 144

Daffodil, 196
Daphne, 197
Death camas, 197
Debris
  in ears, 99
  in eyes, 83, 157
DEET, 178. *See* poisoning general
  procedures, 176-177
Dehydration
  and burns, 70
  and diarrhea/soft stools, 270
  and weakness, 172
Deliveries of kittens, 282
Delphinium. *See* larkspur, 210
Dental disease, 261
Depression, 172
  See also poisonous plants
Detergents, 178. *See* poisoning
  general procedures, 176-177
Devil's ivy. *See* philodendron, 220
Diarrhea, 79-80, 152-153, 270-271
Dieffenbachia. *See* dumb cane, 198
Diesel fuel, 252
Dietary changes
  and diarrhea, 79, 152
  and vomiting, 131
Difficult breathing, 142-143
  normal respiration, 300
Digestive upset, 81-82
Digitalis. *See* foxglove, 202
Dilated pupils. *See* poisonous plants,
  182-231
Discharge
  from ears, 99
  from vulvar area, 129
  from wound, 54
Diseases
  becoming emergencies, general
    information, 260
  cancer, 265

chronic, 267
dental, 261
heart, 89
preexisting and emergency
    treatment, 27
See also vaccinations
Disembowelment, 154
Disinfectants
    as poisons, 236
    use of. *See* wound care, 33
Dishwasher soap, 236
Disorientation
    and head tilt, 158
    and inner ear disease, 99
    and insect ingestion, 100
    and smoke inhalation, 113
    See also poisonous plants
Dizziness. *See* loss of balance, 163
Dracaena palm. *See* corn plant, 193
Dragon tree. *See* corn plant, 193
Drain cleaners, 178, 236
Drooling, 155-156
Drowning, 40
Drugs
    overdose. *See* poisoning general
        procedures, 176-177
    reactions, 144, 166
Dry heaves and toads, 123
    See vomiting, 131
Dumb cane, 198
Dye removers, 236

Ear mites, 168
ears
    blistered, 87
    frostbite, 87
    inner ear disease, 99
    red, 87
    scratching, 168
Easter lily, 198
Eating
    inability to self-feed/head tilt, 58
    See dental disease, 261

See also loss of appetite
Eggplant, 199
Elaine codiaeum, 199
Electric shock
    and burns, 71
    CPR, 40
Elephant's ear, 199
Elizabethan collar
    construction of, 47-49, *illus. 48,
        49*
    purpose of, 47
    See also bite wound abscess,
        protruding organs, skin
        irritations
Emerald feather. *See* asparagus fern,
    231
Emergency
    basic steps, 18
    how to approach, 17-18
    preparing for, 14-18
    techniques. *See* first-aid
        techniques, 29-49
    worksheet, 299
Emergency care, basic steps, 18
Emergency phone numbers,
    identification of, 16, 17
Emergency treatment
    and preexisting diseases, 27
    of kittens, 26
    of older cats, 26
    techniques in. *See* first-aid
        techniques, 29-49
Emergency worksheet, 299
English ivy, 200
Ethanol, 178. *See* poisoning general
    procedures, 176-177
Ethylene glycol, 245-246
Excitability
    and chocolate ingestion, 72
    See poisonous plants, 182-231
Exhaustion
    and strychnine poisoning, 121,
        256

317

See weakness, 172
Exotica perfection dieffenbachia. *See*
dumb cane, 198
Exposure to cold
and frostbite, 87
and hypothermia, 95
providing shelter, 9
External parasites, 274-279
fleas, 274
lice, 277
ticks, 278
Eyes
emergencies, 83
involuntary movement, 99
popped-out, prolapsed, 83
protruding, 103, 164
red, 83
runny, 157-158
scratched, 83
sore, 157-158
tearing, 83, 211

Fava bean, 201
Fecal exam, 273, 304
Feces
bloody, 76
blue-green, 105, 253
examination of, 273, 304
Feeding orphaned kittens, 286
Feline distemper, 302
Feline immunosuppressive virus
(FIV), 27, 301
Feline infectious peritonitis (FIP),
302
Feline leukemia, 27, 301
Feline rhinotracheitis, 302
Fertilizers, 132
Fever
and abscesses, 54
and aspirin ingestion, 63, 242
and infections, 263
and precatory bean ingestion, 222
and spider bites, 119

normal temperature, 300
Fiddle-leaf fig, 201
Finger cherry, 201
FIP, 302
Fire
See burns, 70
See smoke inhalation, 113
First-aid, general instructions, 17-18
First-aid kit, 14-16
list of supplies, 15-16
First-aid techniques
bleeding control, 31-32
cardiopulmonary resuscitation
(CPR), 40-43
Elizabethan collar, 47-49
inducing vomiting, 30
introduction to, 30
muzzle, 44-46
monitoring vital signs, 37-38
wound care, 33-34
wrapping a wound, 35-36
FIV, 27, 301
5-fluorouracil, 178. *See* poisoning
general procedures, 176-177
Flea control products, 247
Fleas, 274-276, *illus. 276*
Floor polish, 236
Floor wax, 236
Florida beauty. *See* corn plant, 193
Fly, ingestion of. *See* insect
ingestion, 100
Foot-pad injury, 159
Foreign objects
choking, 73-75, *illus. 75*, 145-147
protruding from rectum, 76
removal of, from mouth, 73-74,
illus. 75, 145-147
See also prevention of
emergencies, vomiting
Formula for kittens, recipes, 286
4-animopyridine, 178. *See* poisoning
general procedures, 176-177
Foxglove, 202

318

Fractures, 85-86
Frostbite, 87-88
Fruit-salad plant. *See* philodendron, 220
Fur balls. *See* hair balls, 78, 131, 145, 151, 171, 288-289
Fur loss. *See* hair loss, 53, 58, 66
Furniture polish, 236, 252
Furniture wax, 236

Gasoline, 252
German ivy. *See* cineraria, 192
Giant dumb cane. *See* dumb cane, 198
Giardia, 272
Glacier ivy. *See* English ivy, 200
Glue, 178. *See* poisoning general procedures, 176-177
Gold dieffenbachia. *See* dumb cane, 198
Gold dust dracaena. *See* corn plant, 193
Golden pothos. *See* philodendron, 220
Grass, 76
   See also yard chemicals
Green gold nephthytis. *See* philodendron, 220
Ground cherry, 204
Gums
   blue-tinged, 89, 102, 113, 123
   pale or white, 60, 93, 102, 105, 113
   purple, 93, 102, 113
   recessed, 261
   red, 261
   See poisonous plants, 182-231
   yellow, 195
   See also dental disease

Hair loss
   and abrasions, 53
   and allergies, 58

and bite wounds, 66
Hairballs, 78, 131, 145, 151, 171, 288-289
Hairball laxative, 78, 151, 289
Hallucinations and morning glory ingestion, 216
Hazards
   indoors, 8-11
   outdoors, 8-9, 11-12
Head tilt, 158
Health checklist, 306-310
Heart disease, 89-90
Heart failure
   and chocolate, 72
   See heart disease, 89-90
   See poisonous plants, 182-231
Heart rate
   increased and snail bait poisoning, 116, 255
   irregular. *See* poisonous plants, 182-231
   normal, 300
   slow. *See* poisonous plants, 182-231
Heat periods, 288-289
Heat stroke, 91-92
Hemlock, 204, 228
Hemorrhage
   control of, 31-32
   internal and rat poison, 105, 253
   See also bleeding
Herbicides
   and arsenic, 240
   yard chemicals, 132
Hernia, protruding, 103
High-rise syndrome, 8
Hit by car, 93-94
   See also bleeding, fractures, wound care, wrapping a wound
Hives, 144
Holly, 205
Hookworms, 272
Hornets. *See* bee stings, 65

319

Horse bean. *See* fava bean, 201
Horsehead philodendron. *See*
  philodendron, 220
Hospitalization, 290-291
Hot area, 54
Household cleaners, 236
Human medication and cats, 11, 12
  acetaminophen (Tylenol®), 56
  aspirin, 63
  ibuprofin, 97
  See also poisons, list of common
Humane societies and lost cats, 293
Hurricane plant. *See* philodendron,
  220
Hydrangea, 205
Hydrocarbons, chlorinated, 178
Hydrochloric acid, 236
Hyperthermia, 91-92
Hypothermia, 95-96

Ibuprofin, 97-98, 248-249
Illnesses
  in kittens, signs of, 287
  long-term, 267-268
  See also diseases
Inability to lie down and lung disease,
  102
Inability to self-feed and head tilt, 158
Indoor cats, 8-11
Identification tag, 8
Indian laurel. *See* fiddle-leaf fig, 201
Indian tobacco, 206
India rubber plant. *See* fiddle-leaf fig,
  201
Inducing vomiting, 39
Infections, 263
  and dental disease, 261
  prevention of and vaccinations,
  302
  See also bite wound abscesses
  and wound care
Injured cat
  approaching, 20

restraining, 19-21
Inner ear disease, 99
Insect bites
  See bee stings, 65
  See spider bites, ant bites and
  scorpion stings, 119-120
Insect ingestion, 100-101
Insecticides, 132, 256
Insulin, 178. *See* poisoning general
  procedures, 176-177
Internal bleeding, 67-68, 105, 195
Internal injuries
  and bleeding, 67-68
  and fractures, 85-86
  See hit by car, 93-94
Intestinal parasites, 272-273
Iris, 206
Irritated skin, 166-167
  plants causing irritations, 231
Isopropanol, 178. *See* poisoning
  general procedures, 176-177
Itching, 58, 166
Ivermectin, 178. *See* poisoning
  general procedures, 176-177

Janet Craig dracaena. *See* corn plant,
  193
Japanese yew, 207
Jaundice and cycad ingestion, 195
Java bean, 207
Jerusalem cherry, 208
Jessamine, 208
Jimsonweed, 209
Jonquil, 209

Kalanchoe, 210
Kaopectate®
  and diarrhea, 79, 152
  and digestive upset, 81
Kerosene, 252
Kidney
  disease and ibuprofin ingestion, 97
  failure and antifreeze ingestion, 61,

238

failure and plant ingestion. *See* poisonous plants, 182-231

Kittens
birth of, 282, *illus. 284*
feeding, 286-287
illnesses, signs of, 287
orphaned, 285-287
vaccinations, 302-303

Lacerations
and bleeding, 134-135
repair of, 69, 135
Lack of awareness and seizures, 107
Lacy tree philodendron. *See* philodendron, 220
Lameness, 159-160
Larkspur, 210
Laurel, 211
Lead, 250-251
Leukemia, feline, 27, 301
Lice, 277, *illus. 277*
Licking, 70
Lighter fluid, 252
Lightning bug, ingestion of. *See* insect ingestion, 100
Lily of the valley, 211
Limonene, 178. *See* poisoning general procedures, 176-177
Limping. *See* lameness, 159-160
Listlessness, 56, 60, 132
See also weakness/depression, 172
Litter box habits, 161-162
Liver disease
and ibuprifin toxicity, 97
See poisonous plants, 182-231
Loco weeds, 212
Loss of appetite
and abscesses, 54
and anemia, 60
and cancer, 265
and digestive upset, 81

and infections, 263
and uterus infection, 129
and vomiting, 131
and yard chemicals, 132
Loss of balance, 163
Loss of bladder control, 107
Loss of bowel control, 107
Loss of coordination, 163
Loss of hair
and abrasions, 53
and allergies, 58
and bite wounds, 66
Lost cat, 292-293
information form, 296
LSD-like compounds, 216
Lumps, 144
Lupines, 212
Lye, 236

Madagascar dragon tree. *See* corn plant, 212
Manchineel, 213, 231
Marble queen, 213
Marijuana, 213
May apple, 214
Medical health record, 297
Medicine plant, 214
Meowing, distressed
and seizures, 107
and urinary-tract problems, 127
and heat periods, 288
Mercury, 178. *See* poisoning general procedures, 176-177
Metal cleaner, 236
Metal polish, 236
Metaldehyde, 116, 255
Methanol, 178. *See* poisoning general procedures, 176-177
Methylxanthines, 178. *See* poisoning general procedures, 176-177
Milk, digestive problems, 13
Milk-of-Magnesia®, 236
Mineral spirits, 252

321

Missing hair
   and abrasions, 53
   and allergies, 58
   and bite wounds, 66
Mistletoe, 215
Monitoring vital signs, 37-38
Monkshood, 215
Monstera deliciosa. *See*
   philodendron, 220
Morning glory, 216
Moth, ingestion of. *See* insect
   ingestion, 100
Mother-in-law plant. *See* dumb cane,
   198
Mouth irritation. *See* poisonous
   plants, 182-231
Muscle
   contractions and spider bites, 119
   pain and spider bites, 119
   tremors and chocolate, 72
   See poisonous plants, 182-231
Mushrooms, 216
Muzzle
   construction of, 44-45, *illus. 45*
   purpose of, 21, 30, *illus. 46*

Naphthaline, 178. *See* poisoning
   general procedures, 176-177
Narcissus, 217
Narcotic analgesics, 178. *See*
   poisoning general procedures,
   176-177
National Animal Poison Control
   Center, 15, 177
Nausea
   and choking, 145
   and drooling, 155
   and vomiting, 131
Needlepoint ivy. *See* English ivy,
   200
Nervousness
   and chocolate, 72
   and strychnine, 121, 256

Neutering, 303
Nightshade, 217
Nitric acid, 236
Nonpoisonous plants, 232
Nuprin®. *See* ibuprofin, 97
Nutrition, 12-13

Obesity and disease, 27
Oleander, 218
1080, 178. *See* poisoning general
   procedures, 176-177
Onion, 218
Orphan kittens, 285-287
Outdoor cats, 8-9; 11-12
Overdose. *See* poisoning general
   procedures, 176-177
Oxalic acid, 236

Painful areas
   and abrasions, 53
   and allergies, 58
   and bite wounds, 66
   and spider bites, 119
Paint thinner, 252
Paleness and spider bites, 119
Panda. *See* philodendron, 220
Panleukopenia, 302
Panting
   and lung disease, 102
   and smoke inhalation, 113
   See also breathing difficulties
Paper clip, ingestion of
   and choking, 73
   See also foreign objects,
   prevention of emergencies
Paralysis
   and ant bites, 119
   and snake bites, 117
   and spider bites, 119
   See also poisonous plants
Parasites
   external, 274-279
   intestinal, 272-273

322

Pawing
    at eyes, 83
    at mouth, 73, 123
PCP, 178. *See* poisoning general
    procedures, 176-177
Pea, 219
Peace lily. *See* philodendron, 220
Pencil cactus, 219
Peony, 220
Permanent wave neutralizer, 236
Pesticides, 132, 240
Pet carriers
    use of, 23-25
    construction of, 25
Petroleum distillates, 252
Phenols, 178. *See* poisoning general
    procedures, 176-177
Phenylpropanolamine, 178. *See*
    poisoning general procedures,
    176-177
Philodendron, 220
Physical examination, 305-310
Pine oil, 178. *See* poisoning general
    procedures, 176-177
Pins, ingestion of
    and choking, 73
    See also foreign objects,
        prevention of emergencies
Plaque, 261
Plants
    nonpoisonous, 232
    poisonous, 182-231
    skin irritation, 231
    See also specific plant names
Plumosa fern. *See* asparagus fern,
    231
Poinsettia, 221, 231
Poison basics, 175-179
Poisons
    general procedures, 176-177
    list of, 178-179
    poisonous plants, 181-231
    poisons, 232-258

Poisonous plants, 181-231
    See also specific plant names
Pokeweed, 221
Pot belly, 272, 287
Potassium hydroxide, 236
Potato, 222
Pothos. *See* philodendron, 220
Precatory bean, 222
Prevention of emergencies, 8-13
Preventive care, 301-304
    checklists, 10-13, 306-310
    indoors, 8-11
    outdoors, 11-12
    physical exam, 305
Preventive medicine, 12
Preventive nutrition, 12-13
Primrose, 223, 231
Privet, 223
Propranolol, 178. *See* poisoning
    general procedures, 176-177
Protozoa, 272
Protruding eye, 164
Protruding organs, 103-104
Protruding rectum, 165
Pulse
    accelerated, 89
    irregular, 196, 211
    monitoring of, 38
    normal, 300
    slow, 89, 211
    weak, 89, 110
Puncture wound, 54
Pupils
    constricted and plant ingestion,
        206, 216
    dilated. *See* poisonous plants,
        182-231
Pus and blood, 54, 136
Pyrethrins, 179. *See* poisoning general
    procedures, 176-177

Rabies, 155, 302
Raid®, 252

Rapid breathing, 119
normal respiration, 300
See breathing difficulties, 142
See poisonous plants, 182-231
Rashes, 58
See also skin irritations
Rat poison, 105-106, 253-254
Rayless goldenrod, 223
Rectum, protruding, 103, 165
Red emerald. *See* philodendron, 220
Red-margined dracaena. *See* corn plant, 193
Red princess. *See* philodendron, 220
Respirations
monitoring of, 38
normal, 300
See also breathing difficulties, respiratory distress
Respiratory distress, 102
Restlessness, 102
See also anxiety
Restraint techniques, 19-22; *illus. 21-22*
depressed cat, 20
easy-to-handle cat, 20
hard-to-handle cat, 21
Rhododendron. *See* azalea, 185
Ribbon plant. *See* corn plant, 193
Roundworms, 272
Rubber bands. *See* choking, 73
See also foreign objects, prevention of emergencies
Rubbing
eyes, 83
mouth, 123

Sago palm. *See* cycad, 195
Salivation
and arsenic poisoning, 240
and insect ingestion, 100
and spider bites, 119
and toad poisoning, 123
Schefflera. *See* philodendron, 220

Scorpion stings, 119-120
Scrapes. *See* abrasions, 53
Scratching ears, 168
Scratching skin, 166-167
Seizures, 107-109
Shaking
and arsenic poisoning, 240
See poisonous plants, 182-231
Shaking head, 168
Shallow breathing. *See* breathing difficulties, 142
normal respiration, 300
Shivering
and hypothermia, 95
See poisonous plants, 182-231
Shock, 110-112
Skin
abrasions, 53
hardening under, 70
irritations, 58, 119, 132, 166-167, 231, 269
peeling, 70
red, 53, 58, 66
thickening under, 70
Smoke inhalation, 113-115
Snail bait, 116, 255
Snake bites, 117-118
Sneezing, 263
See also breathing difficulties
Snow-on-the-mountain, 225
Sodium carbonate, 236
Sodium hydroxide, 236
Sodium phosphate, 236
Sore
open, 119
weeping, 70
See also bite wound abscess
Spaying, 303
Special considerations, 26
Spider
bites, 119-120
ingestion of. *See* insect ingestion, 100

Splinters, 159
Sprains, 159
Squinting, 83
Staggering
    and arsenic poisoning, 240
    and ibuprofin ingestion, 97, 247
Star-of-Bethlehem, 225
Staples. *See* choking, 73
    See also foreign objects,
        prevention of emergencies
Stiffness and strychnine, 121, 256
Stings
    bee, 65
    scorpion, 119
Stomach, upset. *See* vomiting, 131
    See also abdomen
Stools
    absence of, 78
    black, 195
    bloody, 76, 97, 105, 272
    soft, 270-271
Straining in litter box, 169-170
Stress and lung disease, 102
String
    and choking, 73
    protruding from rectum, 76
    See also foreign objects,
        prevention of emergencies
String of pearls/beads, 226
Striped dracaena. *See* corn plant, 193
Strychnine, 121-122, 256-257
Sulfuric acid, 236
Sweetheart ivy. *See* English ivy, 200
Swelling
    and abscesses, 54
    and bee stings, 65
    and fractures, 85
    and infections, 263
    of ears, 168

Tacks, ingestion of
    and choking, 73
    See also foreign objects,

prevention of emergencies
Tail, severed, 135
Tapeworms, 272
Tarantulas, 119
Taro. *See* elephant's ear, 199
Taro vine. *See* philodendron, 220
Taxus, 226
Teeth, 261
Temperature
    falling
        and shock, 110
        and oleander ingestion, 218
    monitoring of, 37
    normal, 300
    See also fever
Terbutaline, 178. *See* poisoning
    general procedures, 176-177
THC, 178. *See* poisoning general
    procedures, 176-177
Theobromine, 72, 244
Thirst, 61, 97, 129. *See* poisonous
    plants, 182-231
3-IN-ONE® household oil, 252
Ticks, 278-279, *illus. 279*
Tinsel, ingestion of
    and choking, 73
    and protruding from rectum, 76
    See also foreign objects,
        prevention of emergencies
Toad poisoning, 123-124
Toadstools, 227
Toenail, torn, 125-126
Tomato, 228
Tongue, blue-tinged
    and heart disease, 89
    and smoke inhalation, 113
Tooth care. *See* dental disease, 261
Toxins, list of, 178-179
    general procedures, 176-177
    other poisons, 232-258
    poisonous plants, 181-231
Toxoplasmosis, 272
Transporting a cat

325

constructing a carrier, 25
equipment needed, 23
in shock, 24
in stable condition, 24
with back injuries, 24
with fractures, 24
without a carrier, 25
See also fractures, shock
Trash-bag ties, ingestion of
and choking, 73
and protruding from rectum, 76
See also foreign objects,
prevention of emergencies
Tumors, 144, 158
Twitching and seizures, 107
See poisonous plants, 181-231
2,4-D, 178. *See* poisoning general
procedures, 176-177
Tylenol®, 56, 234-235

Urination
and litter box habits, 161
increase of, 97
Urinary-track blockage, 127
Urinary-tract irritations, 127-128
Urine
bloody, 105, 119, 216, 227, 253
dark-colored, 56, 234
red. *See* poisonous plants, 182-
231
Uterus infection, 129-130

Vaccinations, 302, 304
Variable dieffenbachia. *See* dumb
cane, 198
Variegated rubber plant. *See* fiddle-
leaf fig, 199
Vestibular disease, 99
Veterinarian
and emergency care, 17-18
and medication, 56
importance of, 6, 17, 52
Vital signs

decreasing, 110
monitoring of, 37-38
normal, 300
Vitamins and anemia, 60
Vitamin K and rat poison, 105, 253
Vomiting, 131, 171
inducing, 39
See also diarrhea, poisons
Vomitus, blue-green, 105, 253

Wasps. *See* bee stings, 65
Water hemlock, 228
WD-40®, 252
Weakness, 172-173
Weeping fig. *See* fiddle-leaf fig, 199
Whipworms, 272
Wild aconite, 229
Wisteria, 229
Wolf spider. *See* spider bites, 119
Wound care
general, 33-34
wrapping a wound, 35-36
See also abrasions, bite wounds,
burns, lacerations
Wrapping a wound, 35-36
See also abrasions, burns,
fractures, lacerations, skin
irritations, wound care

Xanthine. *See* chocolate, 72, 244

Yard chemicals, 132-133, 258
Yarn
ingestion of and choking, 73
protruding from rectum, 76
See also foreign objects
Yellow jackets. *See* bee stings, 65
Yew. *See* Japanese yew, 207 or Taxus,
226

Zinc oxide, 178. *See* poisoning
general procedures, 176-177